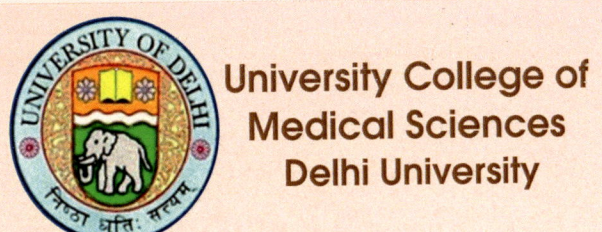

University College of
Medical Sciences
Delhi University

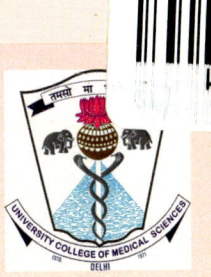

Second Edition

Microbiology
Practical Manual

As per the latest CBME Guidelines

Competency Based Undergraduate Curriculum for the Indian Medical Graduate

Department of Microbiology

Student's Particulars

Name _____

Roll No. _____   Year/Session _____

University Roll No. _____   Name of the Course _____

_____
Signature of Professor and Head

Examiners: _____   _____

Second Edition

Microbiology
Practical Manual

As per the latest CBME Guidelines |
Competency Based Undergraduate Curriculum for the Indian Medical Graduate

Rumpa Saha MBBS MD

Professor
Department of Microbiology
University College of Medical Sciences and GTB Hospital
Dilshad Garden, Delhi

Shukla Das MBBS MD DNB MNAMS

Director-Professor
Department of Microbiology
University College of Medical Sciences and GTB Hospital
Dilshad Garden, Delhi

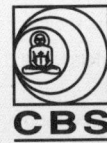

CBS

CBS Publishers & Distributors Pvt Ltd

New Delhi • Bengaluru • Chennai • Kochi • Kolkata • Lucknow • Mumbai
Hyderabad • Jharkhand • Nagpur • Patna • Pune • Uttarakhand

Microbiology
Practical Manual

ISBN: 978-93-54660-68-9

Second Edition: 2022

First Edition: 2020

Published by Satish Kumar Jain and produced by Varun Jain for

CBS Publishers & Distributors Pvt Ltd

4819/XI Prahlad Street, 24 Ansari Road, Daryaganj, New Delhi 110 002, India

Ph: 011-23289259, 23266861, 23266867   Fax: 011-23243014   Website: www.cbspd.com

e-mail: delhi@cbspd.com; cbspubs@airtelmail.in

Corporate Office: 204 FIE, Industrial Area, Patparganj, Delhi 110 092, India

Ph: 011-4934 4934   Fax: 011-4934 4935   e-mail: publishing@cbspd.com; publicity@cbspd.com

Branches

- **Bengaluru:** Seema House 2975, 17th Cross, K.R. Road, Banasankari 2nd Stage, Bengaluru 560 070, Karnataka, India
  Ph: +91-80-26771678/79   Fax: +91-80-26771680   e-mail: bangalore@cbspd.com

- **Chennai:** 7, Subbaraya Street, Shenoy Nagar, Chennai 600 030, Tamil Nadu, India
  Ph: +91-44-26680620, 26681266   Fax: +91-44-42032115   e-mail: chennai@cbspd.com

- **Kochi:** 42/1325, 1326, Power House Road, Opp KSEB, Power House, Ernakulam 682 018, Kerala, India
  Ph: +91-484-4059061-65   Fax: +91-484-4059065   e-mail: kochi@cbspd.com

- **Kolkata:** 147, Hind Ceramics Compound, 1st Floor, Nilgunj Road, Belghoria, Kolkata 700056, West Bengal, India
  Ph: +91-9096713055/7798394118, 9836841399   e-mail: kolkata@cbspd.com

- **Lucknow:** Basement, Khushnuma Complex, 7-Meerabai Marg (Behind Jawahar Bhawan), Lucknow 226001, UP, India
  Ph: 0522-4000032   e-mail: tiwari.lucknow@cbspd.com

- **Mumbai:** PWD Shed. Gala no. 25/26, Ramchandra Bhatt Marg, Next to JJ Hospital Gate no. 2, Opp. Union Bank of India, Noorbaug, Mumbai-400009, Maharashtra, India
  Ph: 022-66661880/89   e-mail: mumbai@cbspd.com

Representatives

• **Hyderabad**	0-9885175004	• **Jharkhand**	0-9811541605	• **Nagpur**	0-9021734563
• **Patna**	0-9334159340	• **Pune**	0-9623451994	• **Uttarakhand**	0-9716462459

Printed at Goyal Offset Workrs Pvt. Ltd., Haryana, India

Foreword

The existence of microorganism was predicted many centuries ago in Jain's literature and by Marcus Terentous Varro in ancient Rome. Louis Pasteur and Robert Koch are the founders of medical microbiology. The life expectancy has increased manyfolds over last 100 years after the development of microbiological techniques. The understanding of microorganisms and microbiological techniques plays an important role for MBBS students in learning the biological basis of disease and its remedies. The learning process has to be gradual, stepwise and crystal clear.

It gives me great privilege to write the Foreword to the book *Microbiology Practical Manual*.

The authors are well known to me for more than a decade and are very motivated and ambitious. They are very experienced in teaching microbiology and are well versed in conducting undergraduate examinations for MBBS students. I have observed keenness and steady craving in them to learn more and endeavour towards perfection. Their eagerness to impart the sound education and create a clinician with clear understanding of the subject is being reflected in developing this manual.

This manual is structured to cover all the practical techniques of microbiology as is being taught and shown to them to achieve uniformity in learning as per the latest CBME guidelines. Hence, it would be of great benefit for microbiology students. I would recommend this manual for all MBBS students.

I congratulate the authors and am delighted to encourage and support them in pursuit of their objective. I wish the authors a grand success.

Dr Anil K Jain
MS FAMS FRCS (Eng.)
Principal
Director-Professor and Head
Department of Orthopaedics
University College of Medical Sciences and GTB Hospital
Delhi

Dr Anil K Jain

Foreword

I am indeed honored to write the Foreword to *Microbiology Practical Manual.* I really appreciate the efforts made by my colleagues Dr Shukla Das and Dr Rumpa Saha for understanding the need of our students and in this endeavor enthusiastically preparing this practical manual as per the latest CBME guidelines.

They are our very dedicated teachers with a deep interest in the subject. As examiners, they are well appreciated by the students.

This manual is very well planned and prepared with the objectives to envelop all the psychomotor domains of undergraduate microbiology and to educate the students to accomplish these tasks with ease. It also aims to attain homogeneous learning. Thus, it would be of definite benefit to microbiology students. I would recommend this manual to all MBBS students.

I applaud the authors and am pleased to encourage them in quest of their objectives. I wish the authors a grand success.

Dr NP Singh
Director-Professor and Head
Department of Microbiology
University College of Medical Sciences and GTB Hospital
Delhi

Preface

*M*icrobiology Practical Manual 2nd edition has been prepared keeping in mind the latest guidelines of Competency Based Undergraduate Curriculum for the Indian Medical Graduate. It provides the Phase II MBBS students relevant, comprehensive, reliable and informative approach to all practical aspects of undergraduate microbiology as per CBME.

This manual contains all images of demonstration slides/specimens and other related items with characteristic features of each, relevant for undergraduate formative training.

For maintaining uniformity, all practical procedures have been clearly written and objectives are defined to enable students to follow and recall.

We express our sincere thanks to our Principal, Director-Professor Dr A K Jain for his encouragement and for writing the Foreword for this manual. Our heartfelt thanks are also for our Head of the Department, Director-Professor Dr NP Singh for his constant support while preparing this manual and writing the Foreword. Thanks are also due to M/s CBS Publishers & Distributors Pvt Ltd for their cooperation and keen interest in the publication of this manual.

Rumpa Saha
Shukla Das

Contents

Section 1: General Microbiology Practicals

Section 2: Perform and Identify the Different Causative Agents of Infectious Diseases by Microscopy

Rules and Safety Precautions to be Observed in the Microbiology Laboratory

1. Wash your hands with soap and water after handling the infectious material.

2. Wear laboratory coats in the laboratory.

3. Keep the nails clean and short.

4. Tie up long hair, while working in the laboratory.

5. Avoid eating, drinking and smoking in the laboratory.

6. Decontaminate the working area with appropriate disinfectant after spillage of potentially infected material.

7. Carry-out the laboratory procedure following standard precautions.

8. Avoid mouth pipetting as far as possible.

9. Perform all the laboratory procedures in a way that minimizes the aerosol formation.

10. Bring practical manual in all the practical classes.

11. Draw properly labeled diagrams neatly, get it corrected from your teachers.

12. Leave your microscope and work seat clean before going out of practical lab.

13. Keep your bag away from working tables.

14. Come exactly at 2.00 pm for practical and tutorials.

Index of Competencies

General Microbiology Practicals

Rules and Safety Precautions to be Observed in the Microbiology Laboratory

1. Wash your hands with soap and water after handling the infectious material.
2. Wear laboratory coats in the laboratory.
3. Keep the nails clean and short.
4. Tie up long hair, while working in the laboratory.
5. No eating, drinking and smoking is permitted in the laboratory.
6. Decontaminate the working area with appropriate disinfectant after spillage of potentially infected material.
7. Carry out the laboratory procedure under sterile conditions.
8. Avoid mouth pipetting.
9. Perform all the laboratory procedures in a way that minimize the aerosol formation.
10. Bring practical manual in all the practical classes.
11. Draw properly labeled diagrams where applicable and get it corrected from your teachers.
12. Leave your microscope and work seat clean before going out of practical lab.
13. Keep your bag away from working tables.
14. Come exactly on time for practical and tutorials.

GLP, Biohazard, Biosafety Levels and Biosafety Cabinets

Good Laboratory Practices

The purpose of good laboratory practice (GLP) is to promote a set of standards for ensuring the quality, reliability, reproducibility and integrity of studies and the reporting of verifiable conclusions and the traceability of data.

Biohazard

Biological hazards or biohazards refer to biological substances that pose a threat to the health of humans. This can include medical waste or samples of a bacteria, viruses, or toxins (from a biological source) that can affect human health or carry significant health risk.

Biohazard symbol is used as a warning symbol for laboratories and those dealing with potentially hazardous material.

Risk groups are classifications that describe the relative hazard posed by infectious agents or toxins in the laboratory. The World Health Organization (WHO) defines the risk groups as:

WHO Risk Group 1 (no/low individual and community risk): A microorganism that is unlikely to cause human disease or animal disease.

WHO Risk Group 2 (moderate individual risk, low community risk): A pathogen that can cause human or animal disease but is unlikely to spread to the community, and effective treatment and preventative measures are available and the risk of spread of infection is limited, e.g. *Staphylococcus aureus*, *Aeromonas hydrophila*, *Corynebacterium diphtheriae*, *Escherichia coli*, *Legionella*, *Sporothrix*, *Microsporum* spp., *Ascaris*, C. *parvum*, herpesviruses, hepatitis viruses.

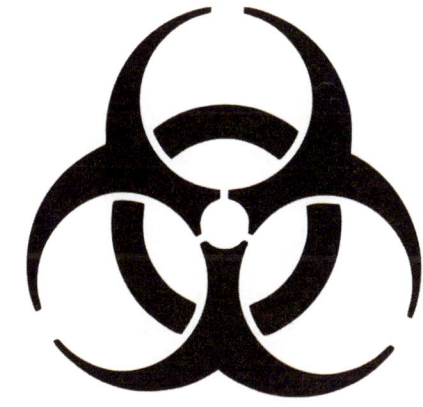

WHO Risk Group 3 (high individual risk, low community risk): A pathogen that usually causes serious human or animal disease and spread from one infected individual to another through inhalation and effective treatment and preventive measures are available, e.g. *Bartonella*, *Burkholderia* spp., M. *tuberculosis*, *Histoplasma*, chikungunya virus, SARS-CoV, yellow fever, prions, HIV.

WHO Risk Group 4 (high individual and community risk): A pathogen that usually causes serious human or animal disease and that can be readily transmitted from one individual to another, directly or indirectly. Effective treatment and preventive measures are not usually available, e.g. Ebola and Marburg viruses, KFD virus, Hendra visus. No bacterial, fungal or parasitic agents fall in this category.

Biological safety levels (BSL) or containment levels are a series of protections designed to safeguards and protect laboratory personnel, as well as the surrounding environment and community. These levels, which are ranked from one to four, are selected based on the agents or organisms that are being researched or worked on in any given laboratory setting.

BSL-1

As the lowest, BSL applies to work with agents on **WHO Risk Group** 1. Research with these agents is generally performed on standard open laboratory benches without the use of special containment equipment. BSL-1 labs are not usually isolated from the general building. There is prohibition of food, drink and smoking materials in lab setting. Personal protective equipment (PPE) is to be worn. Daily decontamination of all work surfaces when work is complete. Infection materials are also decontaminated prior to disposal. Hand washing sink must be available.

BSL-2

This BSL covers laboratories that work with agents **WHO Risk Group 2**. In addition to BSL-1 expectation, the following are to be adhered to appropriate PPE must be worn, including eye protection and face shields. [All procedures that can cause infection from aerosols or splashes are performed within a Class 1 biological safety cabinet (BSC).] A suitable decontamination method is available for proper disposals. The laboratory has self-closing, lockable doors. A sink and eyewash station should be readily available.

Access to a BSL-2 lab is far more restrictive than a BSL-1 laboratory. Outside personnel, or those with an increased risk of contamination, are often restricted from entering when work is being conducted.

BSL-3

Again building upon the two prior biosafety levels, a BSL-3 laboratory typically includes work on WHO Risk Group 2 microbes. The microbes are so serious that the work is often strictly controlled and registered with the appropriate government agencies. Laboratory personnel are also under medical surveillance and could receive immunizations for microbes they work with.

Common requirements in a BSL-3 laboratory include: Standard PPE along with respirators and gowns. All work with microbes must be performed within Class 2 BSC. Access hands-free sink and eyewash are available near the exit. Sustained directional airflow to draw air into the laboratory from clean areas towards potentially contaminated areas (exhaust air cannot be re-circulated). A self closing set of locking doors with access away from general building corridors.

Access to a BSL-3 laboratory is restricted and controlled at all times.

BSL-4

BSL-4 labs are rare. However, some do exist in a small number of places in the US and around the world. As the highest level of biological safety, a BSL-4 laboratory consists of work with highly dangerous and exotic microbes, i.e. WHO Risk Group 4. Examples of such microbes include: Ebola and Marburg viruses.

BSL-4 laboratories have the following containment requirements: Personnel are required to change clothing before entering, shower upon exiting. Decontamination of all materials before exiting. Personnel must wear appropriate PPE from prior BSL levels, as well as a full body, air-supplied, positive pressure suit. A Class III biological safety cabinet is required.

Biosafety level	BSL-1	BSL-2	BSL-3	BSL-4
Description	• No containment • Defined organisms • Unlikely to cause disease	• Containment • Moderate risk • Disease of varying severity	• High containment • Aerosol transmission • Serious/potentially lethal disease	• Max containment • "Exotic," high-risk agents • Life-threatening disease
Sample organisms	E. coli	Influenza, HIV, Lyme disease	Tuberculosis	Ebola virus
Pathogen type	Agents that present minimal potential hazard to personnel and the environment	Agents associated with human disease and pose moderate hazards to personnel and the environment	Indigenous or exotic agents, agents that present a potential for aerosol transmission and agents causing serious or potentially lethal disease	Dangerous and exotic agents that pose a high risk of aerosol-transmitted laboratory infections and life-threatening disease

Biosafety Cabinets

Class I BSC

Room air is drawn in through the front opening and reaches the operator's arms to reach the work surface inside the cabinet while he/she observes the work surface through a glass window. The window can also be fully raised to provide access to the work surface for cleaning or other purposes. The directional flow of air whisks aerosol particles that may be generated on the work surface away from the laboratory worker and is then discharged from the BSC through a high efficiency particulate air (HEPA) filter.

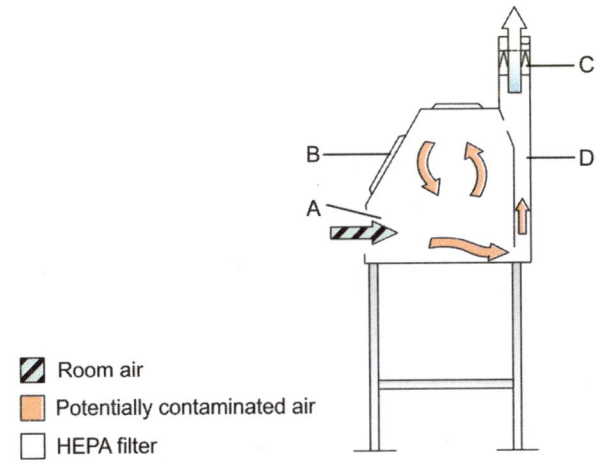

▨ Room air
▨ Potentially contaminated air
☐ HEPA filter

Schematic diagram of a Class I biological safety cabinet.
A. Front opening; B. Sash; C. Exhaust HEPA filter; D. Exhaust plenum.

Class II BSC

It is a ventilated cabinet, which provides personnel, product and environmental protection. It is commonly found in clinical and research laboratories working with infectious agents in Risk Groups 2, 3 and 4 (if positive-pressure suits are used) or with tissue culture.

There are four types (A1, A2, B1, and B2) of Class II BSCs. The main differences between the types are the ratio of air exhausted from the BSC to the air that is re-circulated within the BSC, and the type of exhaust system present.

About 90% of all biosafety cabinets installed are Type A2 cabinets. There is a limited need for Class II Type B BSCs. In addition, Class II Type B BSCs require very specific installation and operating conditions to function correctly.

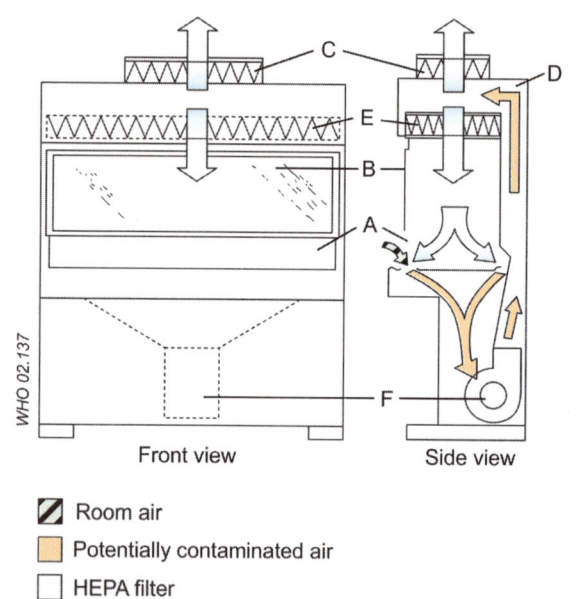

Front view   **Side view**

▨ Room air

▨ Potentially contaminated air

☐ HEPA filter

Schematic diagram of a Class I biological safety cabinet.
A. Front opening; B. Sash; C. Exhaust HEPA filter; D. Rear plenum;
E. Supply HEPA filter; F. Blower.

Class III BSC

This type of cabinet is totally enclosed and is tested under pressure to ensure that no particles can leak from it into the room. Supply air is HEPA-filtered and exhaust air is discharged to atmosphere through two HEPA filters. The operator access the work surface by means of heavy-duty rubber gloves which form part of the cabinet. Airflow is maintained by a dedicated exhaust system exterior to the cabinet, which keeps the cabinet interior under negative pressure.

It may be connected to a double-door autoclave used to decontaminate all materials entering or exiting the cabinet.

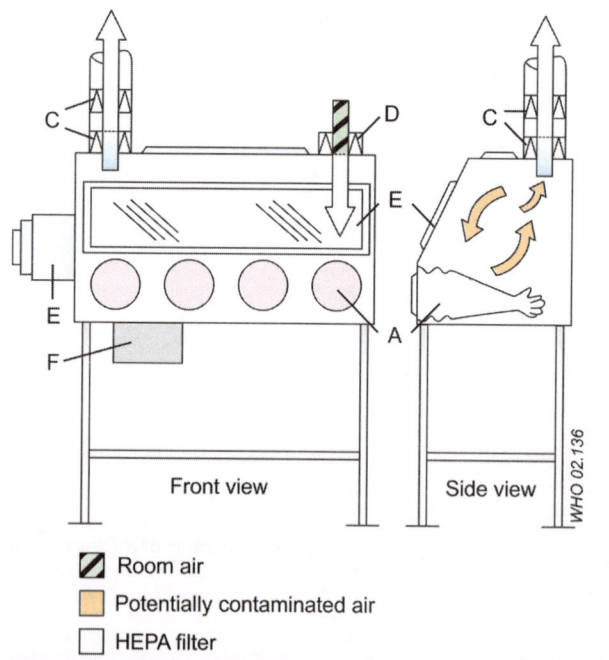

Front view   **Side view**

▨ Room air

▨ Potentially contaminated air

☐ HEPA filter

Schematic diagram of a Class ! biological safety cabinet.
A. Glove ports for arm-length gloves; B. Sash; C. Double-exhaust HEPA filters;
D. Supply HEPA filter; E. Double-ended autoclave or pass-through box; F. Chemical
dunk tank. Connection of the cabinet exhaust to an independent building exhaust air
system is required

BIOSAFETY CABINETS

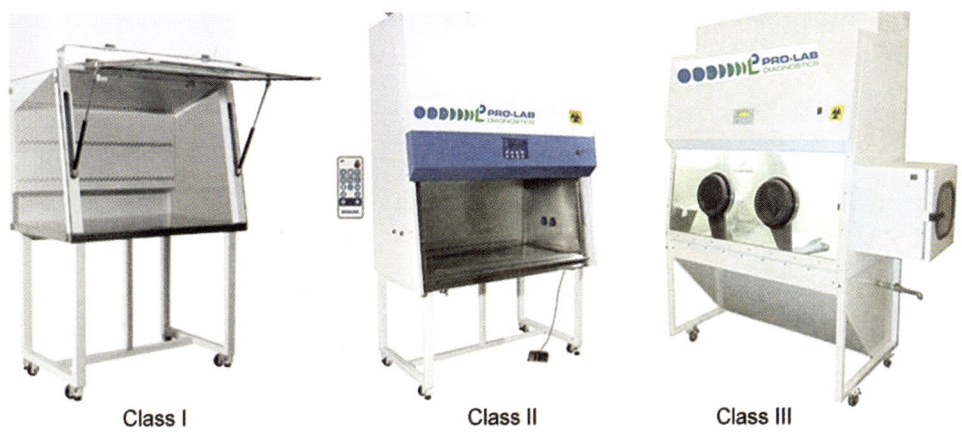

Class I   Class II   Class III

Biosafety cabinets

Features of Class I, II, and III Biological Safety Cabinets (BSCs)

Type	Face velocity (m/s)	Airflow (re-circulated)	Airflow (exhausted)	Exhaust system
Class I	0.36	0	100	Hard duct
Class IIA1	0.38-0.51	70	30	Exhaust to room or thimble connection
Class IIA2	0.51	70	30	Exhaust to room or thimble connection
Class IIB1	0.51	30	70	Hard duct
Class IIB2 (total exhaust BSC)	0.51	0	100	Hard duct
Class III	NA	0	100	Hard duct

Universal Presence of Microbes

Demonstrate the universal presence of microorganisms on animate and inanimate surface.

Method: Using a sterile swab, swab an area on the table top/on hand between the webs of fingers and inoculate on blood agar culture plate. Leave a plate of blood agar exposed in air for 1 hour, cover and incubate the plates overnight by 37°C. Note the growth of microorganisms on the culture plates the next day.

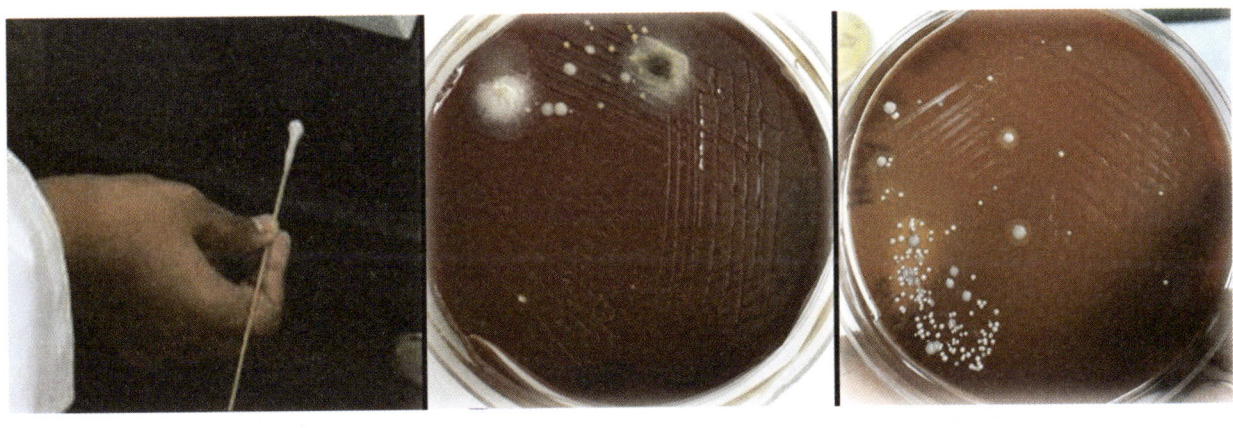

1. On the table top

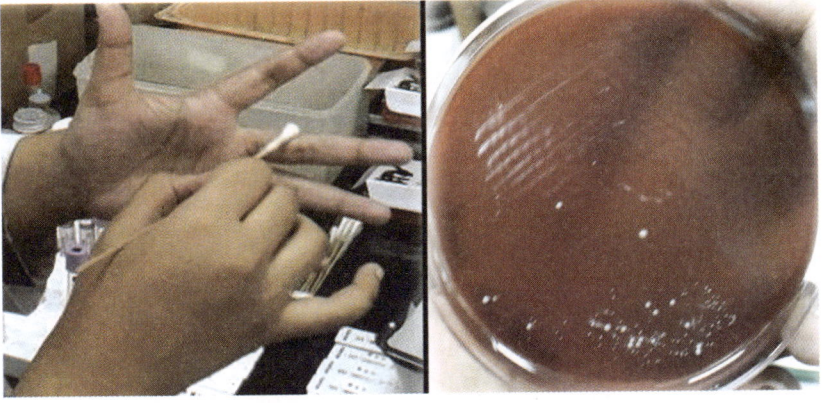

2. Between the webs of fingers

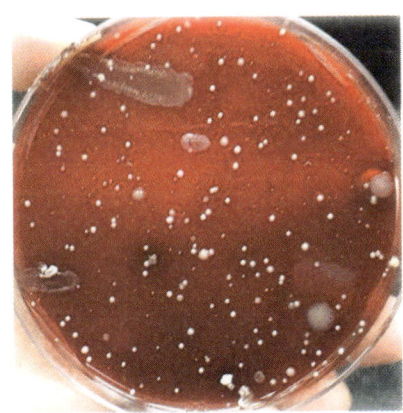

3. From the air after plate is exposed for 1 hour in air

Inference: Microorganisms are present universally.

11

Microscope: General Instructions about Use and Care

1. Always observe an object with the body of the microscope in a perpendicular position. Do not tilt the microscope.
2. Train yourself to look with both eyes open, to reduce eye strain.
3. Do not attempt to take any part of the microscope apart.
4. Use artificial source of light provided on the work table. Use the plain side of mirror.
5. Never leave oil on the objectives. Wipe gently after the use and if oil has been left on for sometime, wipe with lens-paper or soft cloth moistened with xylene.
6. Do not touch the slide with objective lens. Always focus away from the slide, thus avoiding damage to the lens and slide.
7. Partly close the diaphragm for unstained preparation and keep the condenser down.
8. Always focus first with low power and then swing 'high power' in position and bring object into focus with fine adjustment. These two objectives are used for stool, urine, and hanging drop preparations.
9. Oil immersion lens is used for bacterial preparations, etc. Place a drop of oil on slide, lower the lens to touch the oil and focus with fine adjustment. The condenser should be right up when oil immersion is being used.
10. Objectives are as follows:
    • Lower power   – 16 mm
    • High power   – 4 mm focal length
    • Oil immersion – 1.8 mm
    These figures are working distances or focal lengths and very short in the last two, the fine adjustment must be used for focusing.
11. Magnification
    Usual corrected tube length   = 16 cm = 160 mm
    Distance of image   = 16 cm = 160 mm
    Distance of object   = Focal length of objective
    Using low power and eyepiece (EL)—10X

$$\text{Magnification} = \frac{\text{Distance of image}}{\text{Distance of object}} \times \text{Magnification of eyepiece}$$

$$= \frac{160}{16} \times 10$$

12. Always leave your microscope lenses clean, oil and dust-free after you finish your practical.

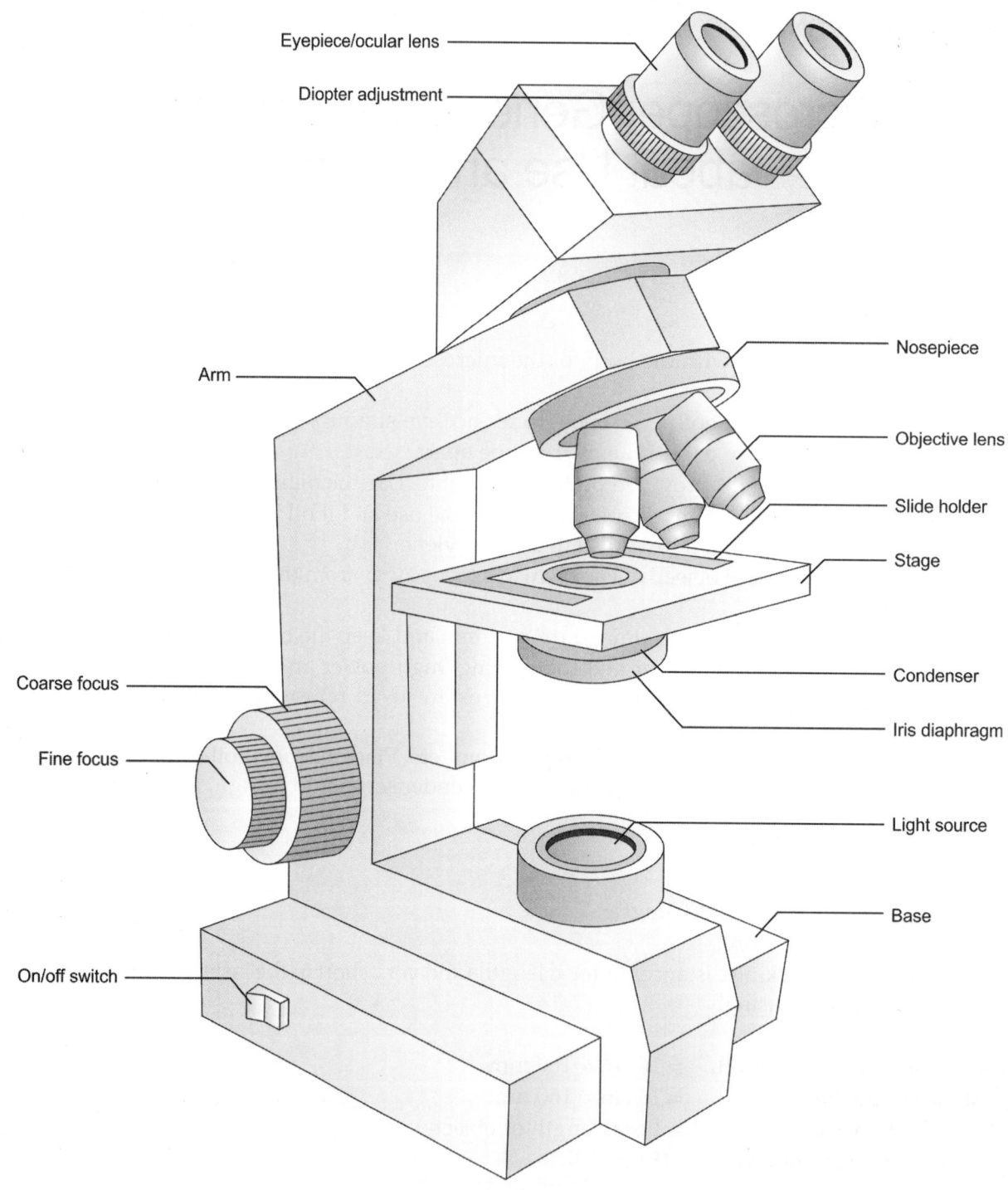

Eyepiece/ocular lens

Diopter adjustment

Arm

Nosepiece

Objective lens

Slide holder

Stage

Coarse focus

Fine focus

Condenser

Iris diaphragm

Light source

Base

On/off switch

Parts of a light microscope

Microscopy and Micrometry

Microscope: Instrument to magnify and resolve microbes and very small objects.

Microscopy: It deals with magnification of object so as to show the finest details of the object.

Principle: The light rays pass through the object, the objective and series of lenses to form a magnified and resolved image of the object. Real, inverted and enlarged image is formed by the objective lens, while virtual erect and enlarged image is formed by eyepiece lens which is seen by the observer.

Parts of a Light Microscope

1. Base—system rests over it.
2. Foot—horseshoe shaped
3. Mirror—directs light in optical system
   Plane mirror to be used for point source of light
   Concave mirror for natural light
4. Condenser—regulates amount of light entering
5. Stage—to place the slide
6. Eyepiece—objects viewed with this
7. Coarse and fine adjustment screw—for focusing clearly and properly.

Position of Condenser

10X: Lowest
40X: Middle
100X: Highest

Types of Microscope

1. **Light/optical microscope:** Uses visible light and a system of lenses to magnify images of small samples.
2. **Phase contrast microscope:** The phase contrast microscope uses the fact that the light passing through a transparent part of the specimen travels slower and due to this is shifted compared to the uninfluenced light. This difference in phase is not visible to the human eye. However, the change in phase can be increased to half a wavelength by a transparent phase-plate in the microscope and thereby causing a difference in brightness. This makes the transparent object shine out in contrast to its surroundings.
   Uses:
   • Identification of cellular structures.
   • Motility of organisms, cell division can be observed in real time.
3. **Darkfield microscope:** The darkfield microscope creates a contrast between the background and the specimen by adding a special stop condenser. The background appears dark and the specimen bright as the stop condenser prevents all the transmitted light reaching the specimen and only the oblique scattered light reaches the specimen and the lens system.

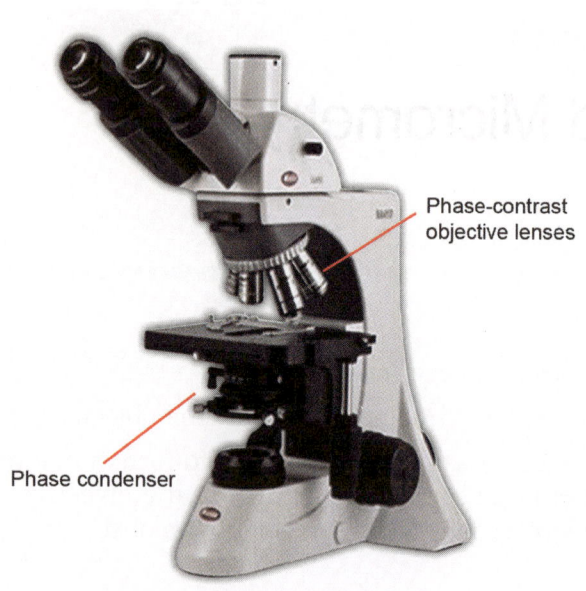

Phase-contrast objective lenses

Phase condenser

Phase-contrast microscope

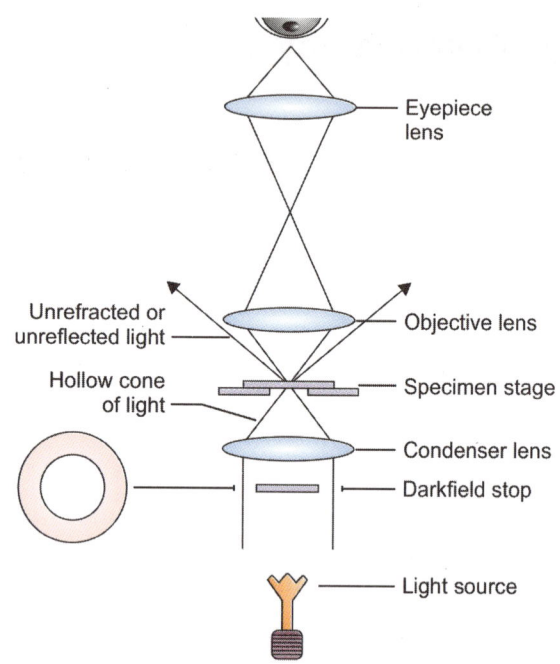

Eyepiece lens

Unrefracted or unreflected light

Objective lens

Hollow cone of light

Specimen stage

Condenser lens

Darkfield stop

Light source

Darkfield microscope

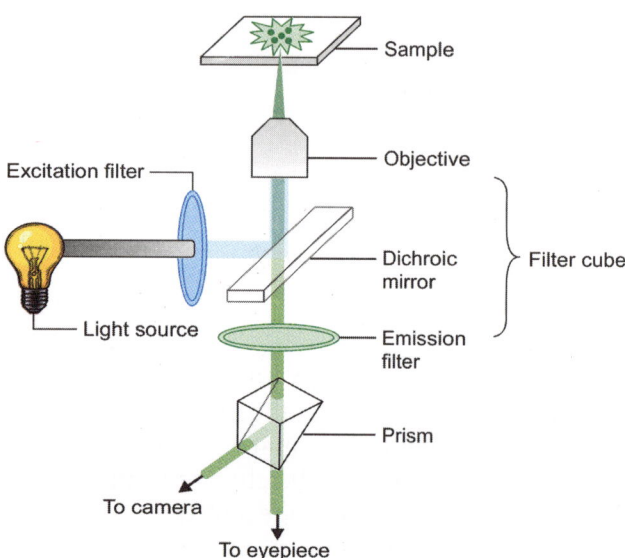

Sample

Excitation filter

Objective

Dichroic mirror

Filter cube

Light source

Emission filter

Prism

To camera

To eyepiece

Fluorescent microscope

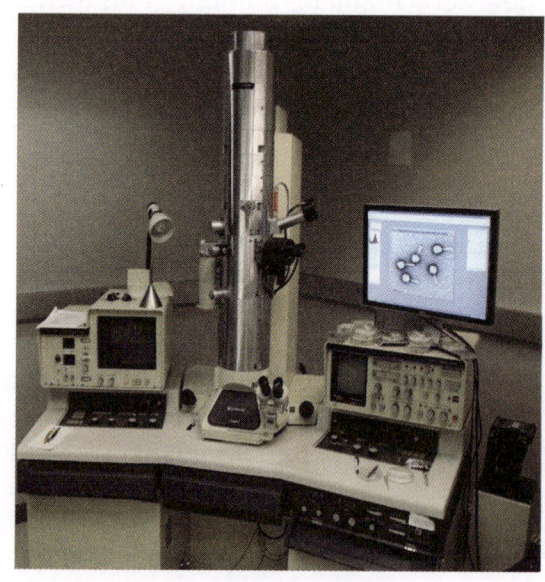

Electron microscope

Uses:
- Identification of treponemas.
- Motility of organisms.
- Observation of thin fragile organisms which cannot be stained.

4. **Fluorescent microscope:** The sample (cells/organism) is stained with a fluorescent dye and UV light source is used. The UV rays passes through the excitation filter and the objective lens on the sample. The reflected higher wavelength wave passes through the beam splitter and emission filter to reach the eyepiece in a fashion that the wavelength of transmitted ray matches the emission characteristics of the fluorescent dye. So, the sample appears colorful on a dark background.
   Uses:
   - Rapid identification of microorganisms, e.g. identification of TB bacilli in sputum, QBC for malaria.
   - Identification of specific protein and DNA in tissue sections.

5. **Electron microscope:** A beam of accelerated electrons is used as a source of light which is passed in a vacuum stack with array of electrostatic and electromagnetic lenses. This beam then passes through the specimen which in part scatters them. This reflected electronic beam carries the structural detail of the specimen and reaches the objective lens which is then further magnified by it. The real image formed is photographically captured and can be seen on a computer screen.
   Uses:
   - High velocity of electrons and low aperture of the EM allow higher magnification up to 0.3–0.5 nm.
   - Visualization of minute cellular detail is possible.
   - Visualization of virus

Micrometry: Measurement of size of microscopic objects is called micrometry.

Basic Principle of Micrometry

Micrometry deals with the measurement of microscopic objects like blood cells, microorganisms, etc. It has two components: The eyepiece micrometer and the stage micrometer.
1. The eyepiece micrometer is a graduated scale from 0 to 10 without standardized measurement.
2. The stage micrometer is a slide with a microscopic 1 mm scale on it. Each division of stage micrometer measures 1/100th mm, i.e. 10 µm (0.001 mm).

After focusing both the eyepiece and the stage micrometer, the scales are aligned and total number of stage micrometer division within 100 divisions of eyepiece micrometer are counted. After this, total length of eyepiece micrometer is calculated and divisional measurement is calculated by unitary method. After obtaining the measurement of single eyepiece division the stage micrometer is removed and the slide with the sample is focused. Number of eyepiece division within a single cell is counted and multiplied by the eyepiece division.

Remarks: The measurement of eyepiece division is not constant and changes with the magnification of the objective and the tube length.

Example: At 40X magnification, 100 eyepiece divisions are equivalent to 25 stage divisions, i.e.

100 eyepiece division × size of each eyepiece division (n) = 25 stage divisions × size of each stage division (10 µm),

$$n = \frac{25 \times 10 \text{ µm}}{100}$$

$$n = 2.5 \text{ µm}$$

Focus a Giemsa stained blood slide and calculate number of eyepiece divisions within a RBC.

Suppose, 1 RBC = 3 eyepiece divisions

Then diameter of 1 RBC = 3 × 2.5 µm = 7.5 µm

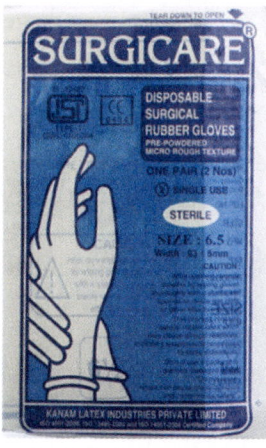

A pair of disposable surgical rubber gloves of size 6.5

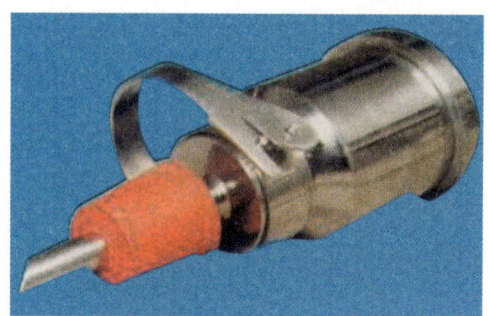

Seitz filter

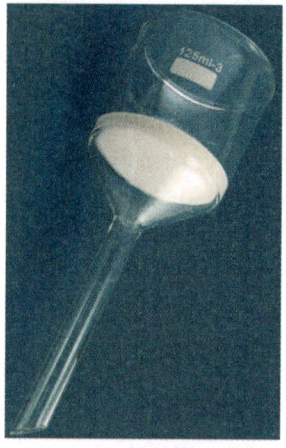

Sintered glass filter

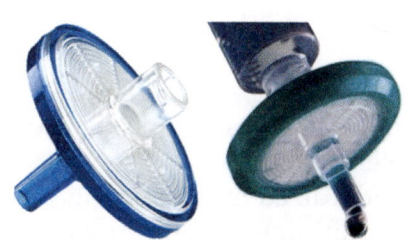

Millipore membrane filter available in pore sizes 0.22 μm/0.45 μm

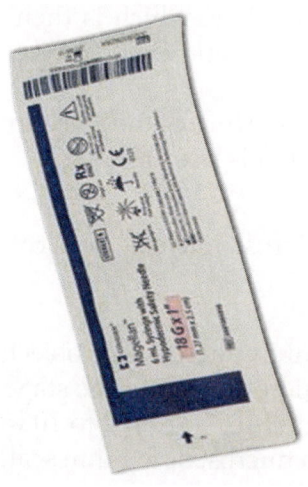

Sterile disposable plastic syringe of 2 ml capacity with 18G hypodermic needle

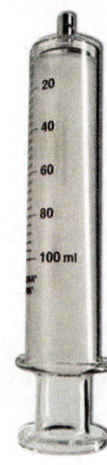

Glass syringe of 100 ml capacity

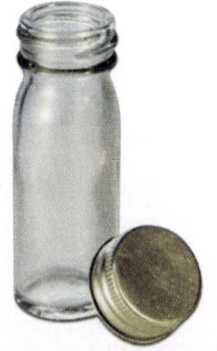

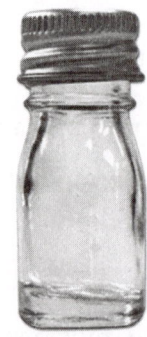

Universal container (McCartney bottle)

Bijou bottle

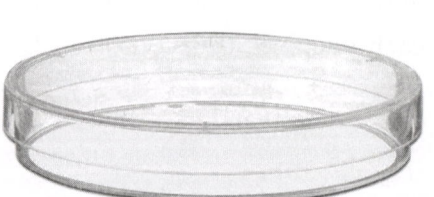

Glass Petri plate

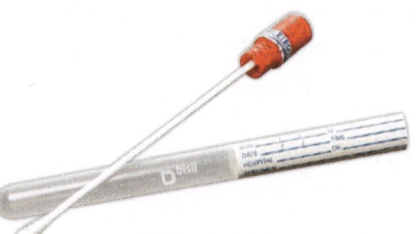

Sterile swab

Methods of Sterilization and Disinfection

METHODS OF STERILIZATION	
METHODS	**EXAMPLE**
PHYSICAL METHODS	
I. HEAT	
1. Moist heat	
a. Below 100°C	Vaccine bath; pasteurization; inspissation
b. At 100°C	Boiling steaming, tyndallization
c. Above 100°C	Autoclave: Dressings, surgical instruments, culture medias
2. Dry heat	
a. Flaming, red heat	Bacteriological loupe
b. Hot air oven scissors, and blades	Lab glass wares, powders, oils; liquid paraffin, glycerol, scalpels,
II. IONISING RADIATION	
Gamma rays	Disposable syringe needles/gloves/catheters/swabs
III. FILTRATION	
1. Seitz filter	Serum, vaccine
2. Sintered glass filter	Serum, vaccine
3. Millipore filter	Serum, vaccine
CHEMICAL METHODS	
Chemicals	Glutaraldehyde
GASEOUS STERILANTS	
Gas: Ethylene oxide (EtO)	Disposable syringe needles/gloves/catheters
Plasma sterilization	Arthroscopes, laparoscopes, spine sets
METHODS OF DISINFECTION	
Alcohols	70% ethylalcohol, isopropyl alcohol
Phenols	Cresol; chlorhexidine, hexachlorophene
Halogens	Sodium hypochlorite, iodine
Aldehydes	Formaldehyde
Antiseptics	Mercuric chloride; acriflavin

LABORATORY AUTOCLAVE

Principle

Water boils when vapour pressure equals that of the surrounding atmosphere. At normal pressure water boils at 100°C. When the atmospheric pressure is raised as in a closed vessel like autoclave, the temperature at which water boils also increases. Steam at higher temperature has a greater penetration power.

Temperature = 121°C;
Time = 15 minutes
Pressure = 15 lbs/square inch

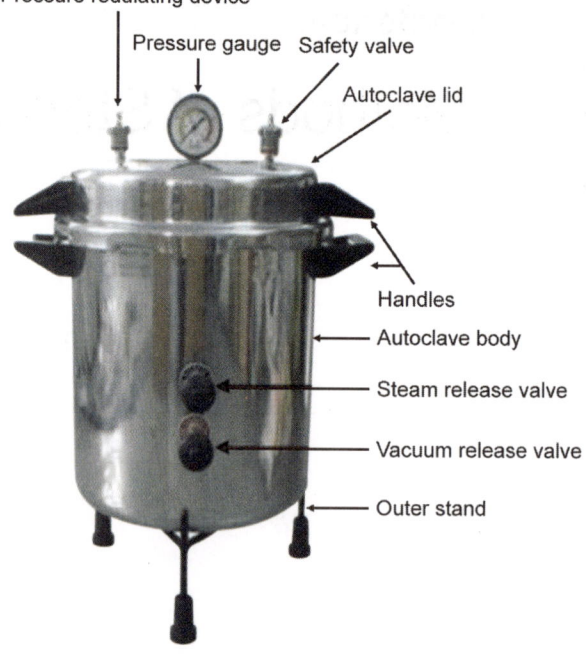

Vertical autoclave

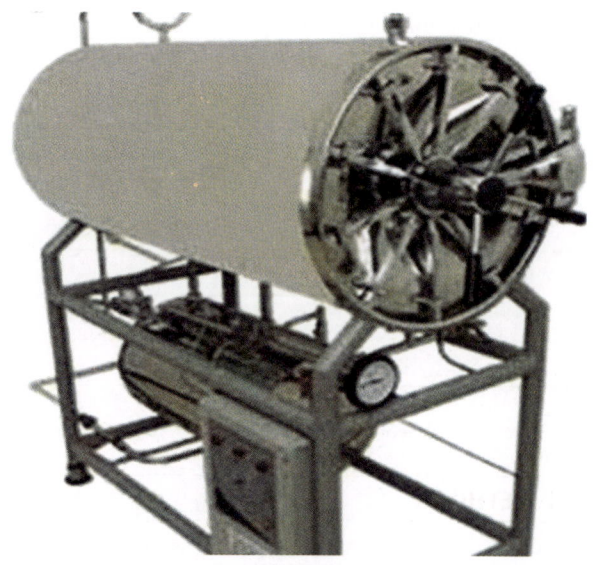

Horizontal autoclave

HOT AIR OVEN

Principle

Hot air ovens are electrical devices which use dry heat to sterilize. Hot air ovens use extremely high temperatures over several hours to destroy microorganisms and bacterial spores. The ovens use conduction to sterilize items by heating the outside surfaces of the item, which then absorbs the heat and moves it towards the center of the item. Generally, they use a thermostat to control the temperature. Their double walled insulation keeps the heat in and conserves energy, the inner layer being a poor conductor and outer layer being metallic.

The commonly used temperatures and time that hot air ovens need to sterilize materials are:

170°C for 30 minutes (1/2 hour)

160°C for 60 minutes (1 hour)

150°C for 150 minutes (2½ hours)

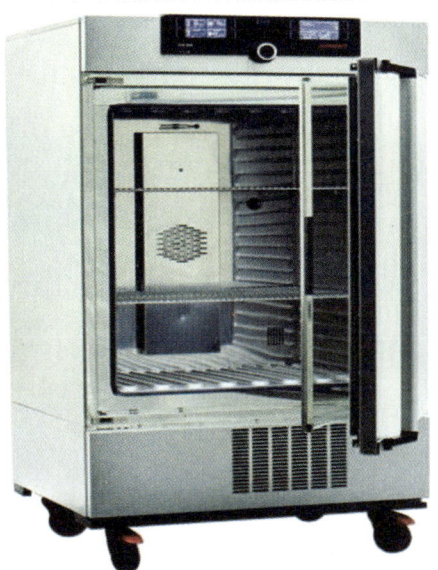

Hot air oven

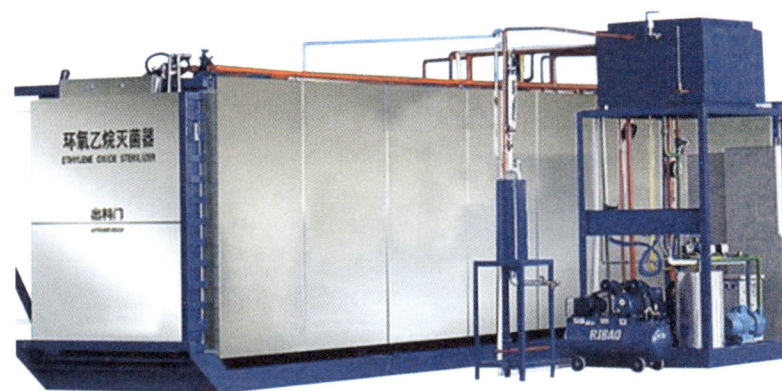

Ethylene oxide (EO) sterilizer

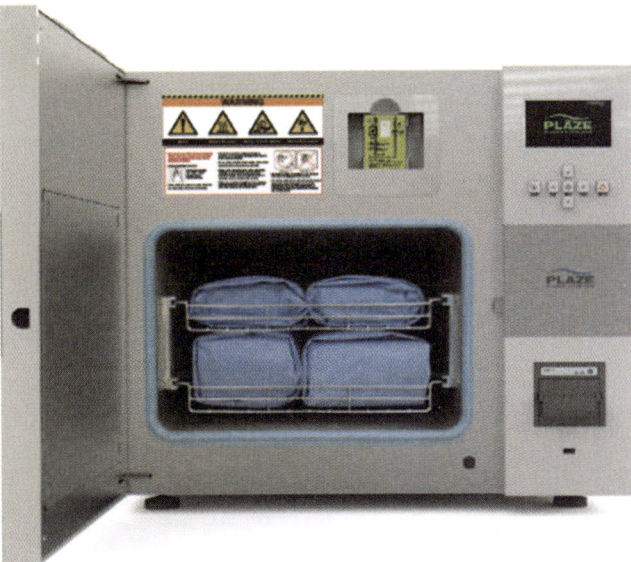

Plasma sterilizer

Biomedical Waste Disposal

DISCARDING HAZARDOUS MATERIAL

Colour Codes for Discard of Biomedical Wastes

(BMW Rules 2016 with Central Pollution Control Board Revision 5)

Category	Type of BMW	Type of bag
Yellow	• Disposable masks • Disposable nonplastic coverall/gown • Shoe covers • Head covers • Wastes contaminated blood/body fluids • Blood bags • Expired/discarded cytotoxic drugs • Discarded/expired vaccines	Yellow colored nonchlorinated plastic bags
Red	• Goggles and face-shields • Gloves • Blood bags • Syringe, IV set, nasogastric tubes, central line catheter • Urine catheter with urobags • Disposable plastic coverall/gown • Used automated blood culture bottles	Red colored nonchlorinated plastic bags
White	• Waste sharps, e.g. needles, scalpels	Puncture proof, leak proof, tamper proof container/box
Blue	• Glassware, e.g. glass ampoules • Microscopy slides • Metallic implants	Puncture proof, leak proof, tamper proof container/box
General green	• Biodegradable general wastes, e.g. leftover food	
General blue	• Nonbiodegradable general wastes, e.g. disposable plates and cutlery	

- All bin should have foot operated lids
- Bin bags should be double layered as to ensure adequate strength and no-leaks
- Collection bin for Covid waste should be labelled as "COVID-19"

Table of Commonly Used Culture Media in Microbiology and their Uses

COMMONLY USED CULTURE MEDIA IN MICROBIOLOGY AND THEIR USES

Name of media	Type of media	Important constituents	Uses
Peptone water	Basal media	1% Peptone NaCl, water	• Sugar fermentation test after addition of 1% respective sugar to peptone water • Sub-culture of bacteria
Nutrient agar	Basal media	Peptone water Meat extract Agar	Growth of nonfastidious bacteria
Blood agar	Enriched media	Nutrient agar 5% sheep blood	Growth of aerobic and anaerobic bacteria
Chocolate agar	Enriched media	Heated blood agar	Growth of fastidious bacteria, e.g. Neisseria
MacConkey agar	Differential media or mildly selective media	Peptone Lactose Bile salt Neutral red (indicator) Agar	Differentiating lactose fermenters (LF) from nonlactose fermenting (NLF) gram-negative bacteria
Loeffler's serum slope	Enriched media	Glucose broth 1 part Serum 3 part	Selective growth of *Corynebacterium diphtheriae*
Tellurite blood agar	Selective media	Blood agar Potassium tellurite (0.4%)	Growth of *Corynebacterium diphtheriae* (black colonies)
Xylose lysine deoxycholate /(XLD) agar	Moderately selective media	Mainly .... Xylose Lysine Na-deoxycholate Phenol red (indicator) Lactose, sucrose, agar	Growth of *Salmonella* spp. (red colonies with black centre) and *Shigella* spp. (red colonies without black centre)
Wilson and Blair bismuth sulphite agar	Highly selective media	Peptone Beef extract Dextrose (glucose) Disodium phosphate Ferrous sulphate Bismuth sulphite Brilliant green (indicator) Agar	Black colonies of *Salmonella typhi*

Contd.

Contd.

Name of media	Type of media	Important constituents	Uses
Löwenstein-Jensen (LJ) medium	Selective media	Hen's egg (solidifying agent) Malachite green (selective agent) L-asperagine Glycerol Mineral salts	Growth of *Mycobacterium TB* (rough, tough, buff) and nontuberculous mycobacteria (yellow)
Thiosulphate citrate bile-salt sucrose (TCBS) agar	Highly selective media	Bile Sucrose Bromothymol blue (indicator) Salts Agar Water	Differentiating *Vibrio cholerae* (yellow sucrose ferming) from *V. parahaemolyticus* (nonsucrose fermenting green colonies)
Müeller Hinton agar	Nonselective Nondifferential medium	Beef infusion Casein Starch Agar Water (cation adjusted)	Antimicrobial sensitivity testing (AST)
Robertson's cooked meat broth	Enriched media	Nutrient broth Cooked meat particles Yeast extract Dextrose	Used for growth of anaerobic organisms
Thioglycolate broth	Enrichment broth	Casein Dextrose, NaCl Yeast Extract Na thioglycollate Cystine, resazurin Agar	Used for growth of anaerobic organisms
Selenite F broth	Enrichment broth	Peptone water Na-selenite	Selective culture of feces to grow fecal pathogens for 4–6 hours followed by SC
Alkaline peptone Water	Enrichment broth	Peptone water at pH 9.0	Selective culture of *Vibrio cholerae* from feces for 4–6 hours followed by SC
Brain heart infusion broth/agar	BHIB-liquid BHIA-solid Biphasic BHIB/A	Calf brain Salts Glucose Agar to solidify	Growth of variety of fastidious and nonfastidious bacteria from blood culture in BHIB
Sabouraud dextrose agar (SDA)	Selective media	Peptone Dextrose 4% Water Agar	Growth of fungi

Demonstration of Common Culture Media and Biochemical Reactions

The following media are commonly used for gram-negative bacilli of the family Enterobacteriaceae.

Blood Agar

- It is an **enriched medium.**
- Contains **5% sheep blood** in nutrient agar.
- Helps to differentiate between **α and β hemolysis.**
- Helps to **study swarming** by *Proteus* spp.
- Preparation: Autoclaved nutrient agar is cooled to 50°C followed by addition of defibrinated sheep blood aseptically.

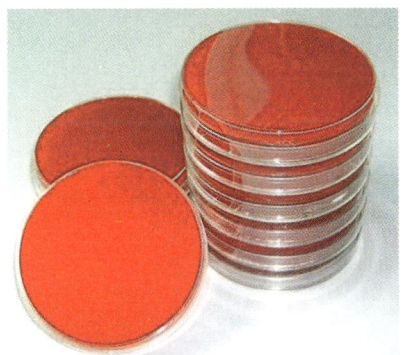 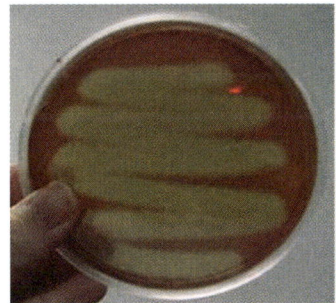 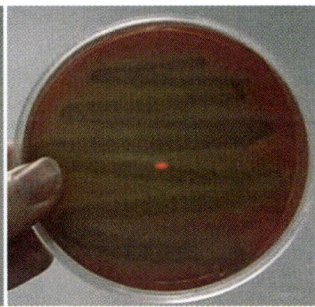

Beta hemolysis   Alpha hemolysis

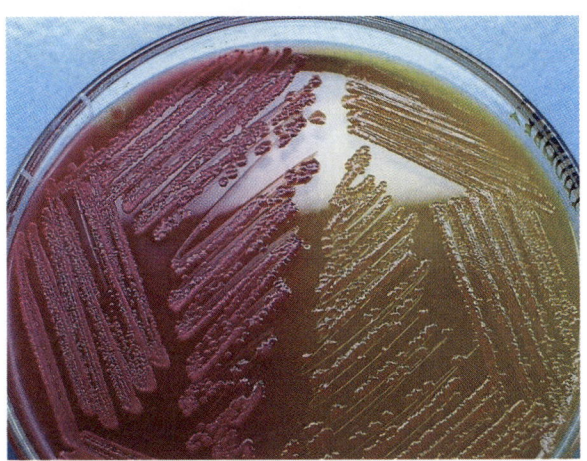

Lactose fermentor colonies   Nonlactose fermentor colonies

MacConkey agar

MacConkey Agar

- It is a **mildly selective media** as it selects out lactose fermenting (**LF) pink colonies** from nonlactose fermenting (**NLF) pale colonies**.
- It is also an **indicator medium** and contains neutral red indicator.
- Contains bile salt (sodium taurocholate) hence **prevents swarming.**

Xylose Lysine Deoxycholate (XLD) Agar

Moderately selective media for:

- *Salmonella* (pink colonies with black centre)
- *Shigella* (pink colonies)

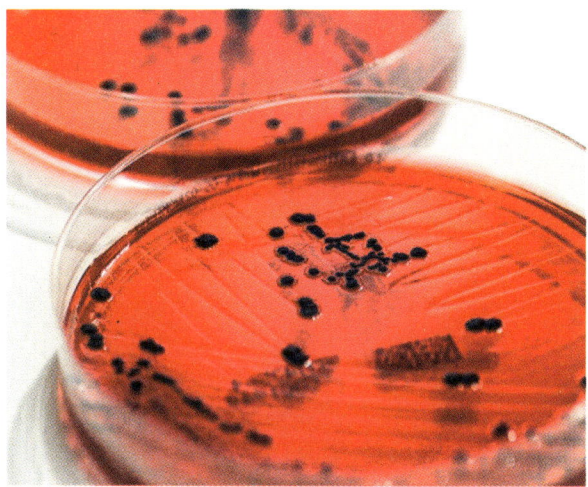

XLD agar

BIOCHEMICAL TESTS

Catalase Test

Principle: Bacteria that produce enzyme catalase breaks down H_2O_2 into H_2O and O_2. The O_2 is released as bubbles.

Reagent used: 3% H_2O_2

A drop of 3% H_2O_2 is put on a glass slide. With a wooden applicator stick bacteria is transferred from fresh culture to H_2O_2 on slide and observed for immediate and sustained bubbles formation.

Catalase producing bacteria: Staphylococcus, all gram-negative organisms of family Enterobacteriaceae.

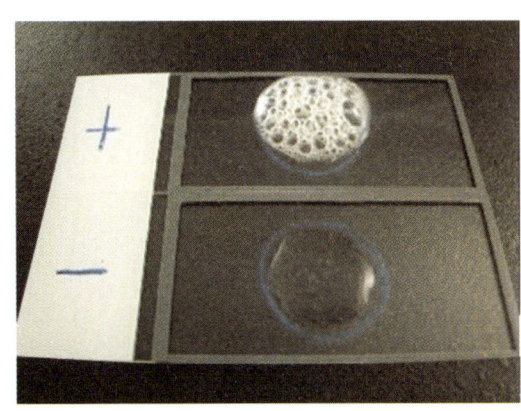

Oxidase Test

Reagent: Tetramethyl *para*-phenylenediamine dihydrochloride.

Test:

- A strip impregnated with the reagent is taken.
- A small portion of the colony is picked-up with the corner of a sterile coverslip and smeared onto the strip.
- Change of color to purple within 30 sec signifies positive reaction.

Principle: The cytochrome oxidase enzyme of certain bacteria is able to oxidize the reagent producing the coloured product.

Example: Positive—*Pseudomomas* spp., *Vibrio* spp.
Negative—members of family Enterobacteriaceae

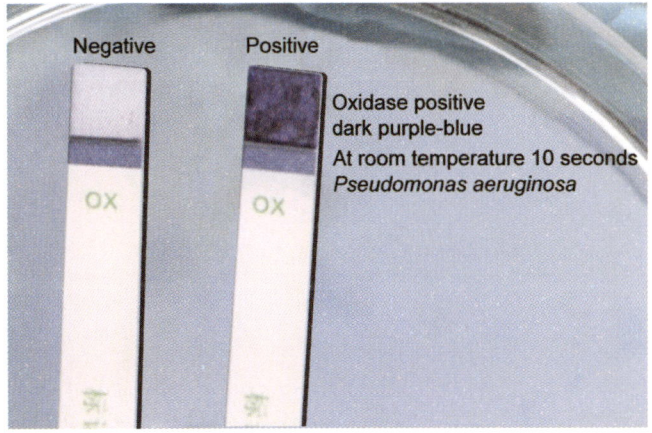

Oxidase test

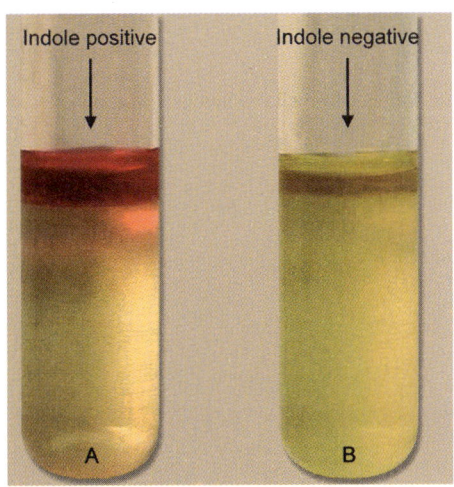

Indole production test

Indole Production Test

- **Principle of test:** Ability of an organisn to split indole from tryptophan.
- **Reagent used:** Kovac's reagent
- **Indole producing organisms:** *E. coli, Proteus vulgaris*.

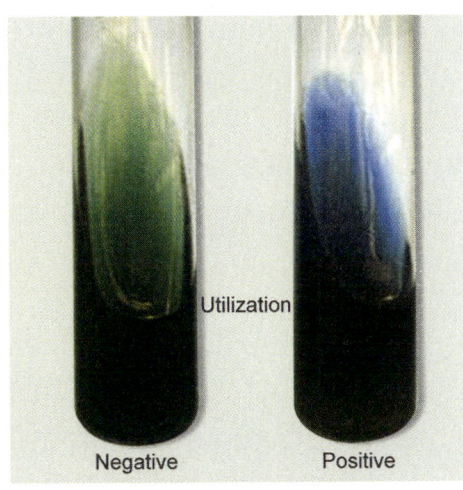

Citrate utilization test

Citrate Utilization Test

- **Principle:** Ability of an organism to utilize citrate as the sole source of carbon for metabolism resulting in alkalinity.
- **Medium:** Simmon's citrate medium
- **Indicator:** Bromothymol blue
- **Citrate utilizing organisms:** *Klebsiella, Salmonella, Enterobacter.*

Urease Production Test

- **Principle:** Ability of an organism to produce the enzyme urease which hydrolyzes urea to ammonia resulting in pink color.
- **Medium:** Christensen's urea agar
- **Indicator:** Phenol red
- **Urease producing organisms:** *Proteus, Providencia, Helicobacter pylori, Klebsiella, Cryptococcus* (yeast fungus)

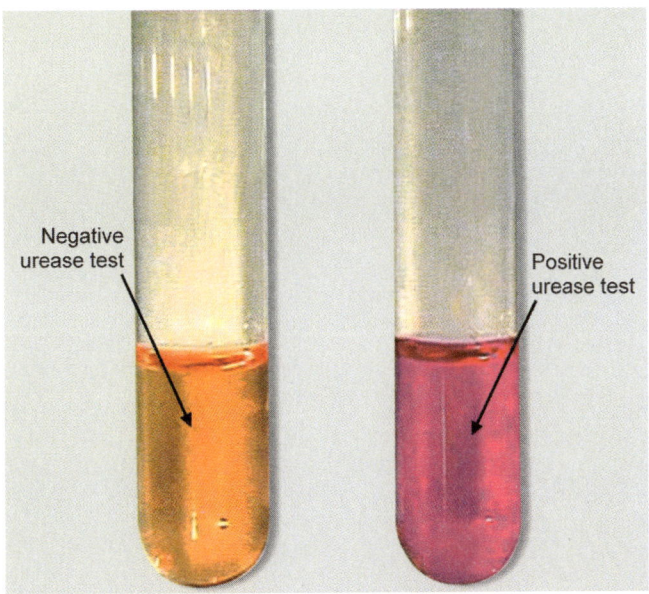

Urease production test

Methyl Red (MR) Test

- **Principle:** Ability of an organism to produce and maintain stable acid end-products from glucose fermentation and overcome buffering capacity of the system.
- **Medium:** Glucose phosphate broth
- **MR positive organisms:** *E. coli*, *Yersinia* spp.

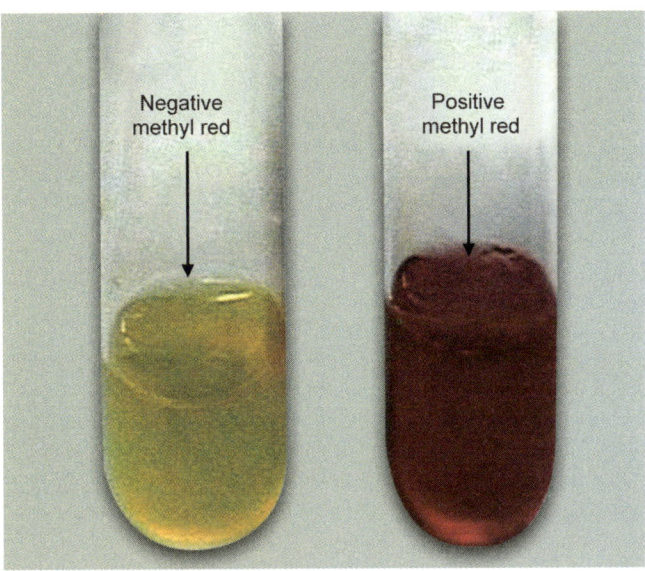

Methyl red test

Voges-Proskauer (VP) Test

- **Principle:** Ability of an organism to produce neutral end product acetylmethylcarbinol/acetoin from glucose fermentation
- **Medium:** Glucose phosphate broth
- **VP positive organisms:** Klebsiella, Enterobacter

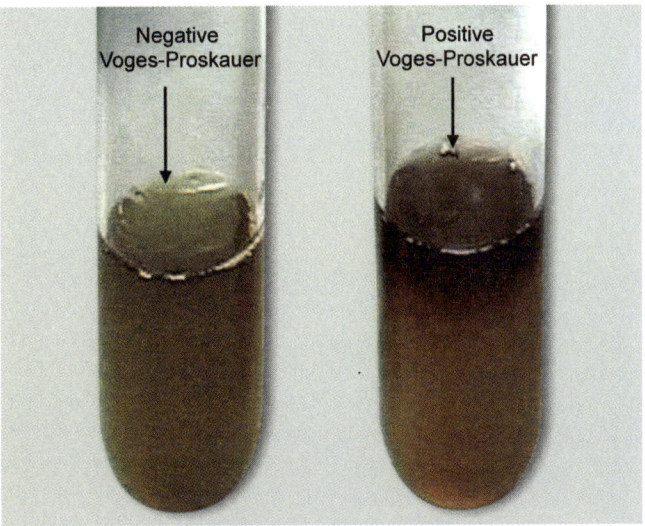

Voges-Proskauer test

Tripple Sugar Iron (TSI) Test

Principle: Tests the production of acid and gas from fermentation of three sugars—lactose, sucrose, glucose (present in ratio of 10:10:1 parts) and also the ability to produce H2S.

Medium: Has a butt and slant. Contains lactose, sucrose, glucose (present in ratio of 10:10:1 parts). Indicator is phenol red.

Interpretation

Glucose fermentation: Acidic (yellow) butt
Sucrose/lactose fermentation: Acidic (yellow) slant
Both glucose and sucrose/lactose fermentation: Acidic (yellow) slant and butt
Gas production: Cracks in medium/medium lifted up
H2S production: Blackening of the medium
No fermentation: Both slant and butt alkaline

Slant/butt	Glucose	Lactose	Sucrose
K/A	+	–	–
A/A	+	+	+/–
K/K	–	–	–

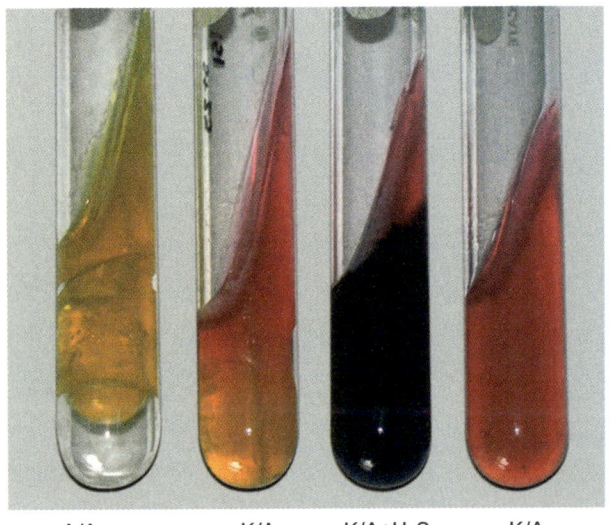

A/A + gas   K/A   K/A+H$_2$S   K/A

Organism	Slant/butt	Gas	H2S
E. coli/Klebsiella	A/A	+	–
Proteus	A/A	–	+
S.typhi	K/A	–	+
Shigella	K/A	–	–
Pseudomonas	K/A	–	–

Culture Methods

The purpose of culture is

- To isolate bacteria in pure form
- To identify the bacteria
- To be able to do antibacterial sensitivity testing
- Demonstrate the properties of the bacteria
- For research purposes
- Maintain a stock of the bacteria

Different methods of culture of bacteria are as follows.

Culture on Solid Medium

1. **Streak culture** which is most commonly used for inoculation of specimens for isolation or for obtaining isolated colonies of different bacteria from a mixed culture.

   A loopful of the specimen is smeared onto the solid media to form an oval shapes well of primary inoculum (A). This is then spread over the media by streaking parallel lines onto the media to form secondary (B) followed by tertiary (C) and subsequent inoculums (D & E) ending in a feathery tail. The loop may be heated in between different set of streaks to obtain isolated colonies which is the target of this type of culture.

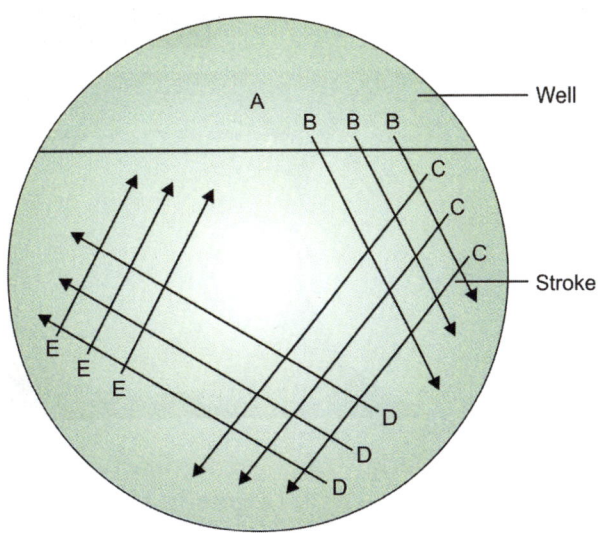

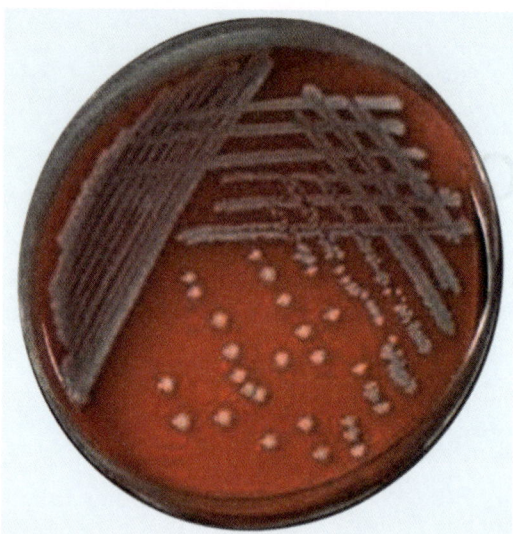

On incubation the growth may be confluent at the original inoculation but becomes progressively thinner and isolated colonies are obtained over the final series of streaks.

2. **Lawn culture or carpet culture** provides an uniform growth of the bacteria for antibiotic sensitivity testing or phage typing. It is prepared by either flooding the culture plate with a pure liquid culture or suspension of the bacterium and then pipetting out the excess inoculum or the surface of the plate may be inoculated by a swab soaked in liquid culture or suspension of the bacterium.

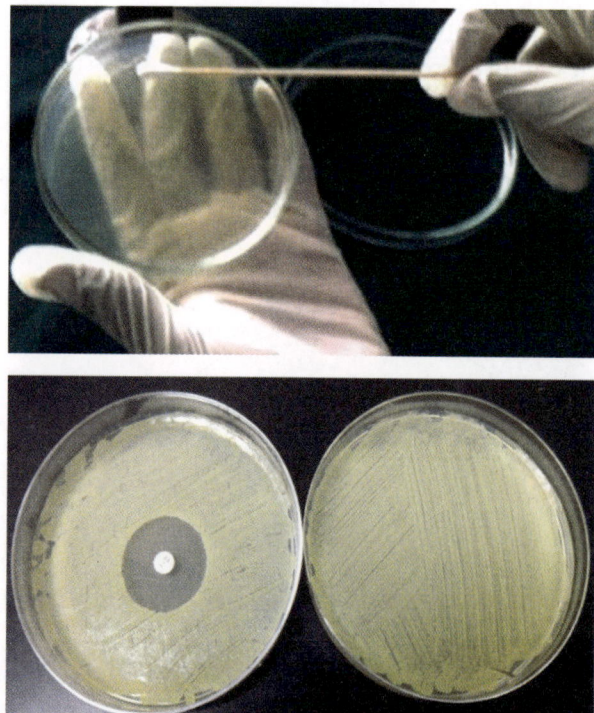

3. **Stab culture** is prepared by charging a long straight wire dipped in a liquid culture and then into a tube of suitable culture medium like nutrient agar or gelatin to demonstrate certain characteristics of the bacterium like motility or gelatin liquefaction.

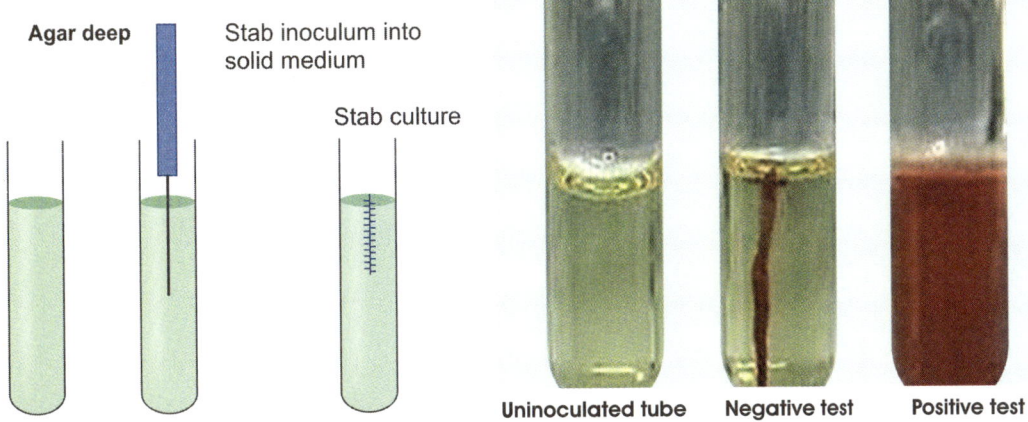

4. **Stroke culture** is made on agar slope or slants in tubes for providing a pure growth of the bacterium for demonstrating certain properties.

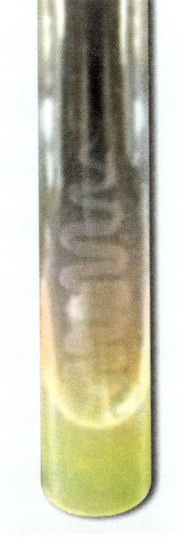

5. **Pour plate culture** is prepared by first melting agar medium with subsequent cooling then adding the bacterial inoculums and then pouring onto a sterile Petri dish and allowing it to set and then after incubation of the plate colonies will be seen well distributed in the depth of the medium. It is used for quantitative urine culture as it gives the viable counts.

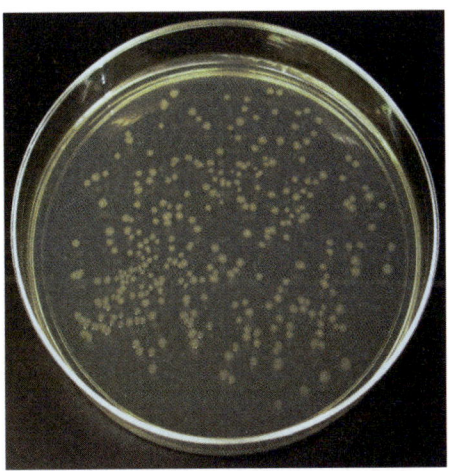

Culture on Liquid Medium

These are inoculated by touching suitable liquid medium with charged loop or straight wire or by adding inoculums with pipettes or syringes. This method is used for blood culture or for preparing inocula containing antibiotics for micro or macro broth dilutional method for antibiotic sensitivity testing.

Description of the Appearance of Growth on Solid or in Liquid Media

Aim: To describe colony characteristics of bacterial growth on solid and lequid media.

Description of Colonies on Solid Media

1.	Name of the media	: Blood agar, MacConkey agar, etc.
2.	Shape	: Circular, irregular, radial
3.	Size	: In millimeters (approx.), pinpoint, pinhead
4.	Elevation	: Raised, low convex, dome shaped, umbonate
5.	Surface	: Smooth, rough, granular, dull or glistening
6.	Edge	: Entire, crenate, spreading
7.	Color	: Colored by reflected and transmitted light, fluorescent
8.	Opacity	: Transparent, translucent or opaque
9.	Consistency	: Butyrous/mucoid/friable
10.	Emulsifiability	: Easy or difficult
11.	Pigment	: Pigmented—diffusible or nondiffusible/nonpigmented
12.	Change in medium	: Haemolysis on blood agar
13.	Odor	: Present seminal/fishy/earthy or absent

Growth in Liquid Medium

1.	Degree	: None/scanty/moderate/abundant
2.	Turbidity	: Present or absent
3.	Deposit	: Present or absent
4.	Surface pellicle	: Present or absent
5.	Odor	: Absent or fishy/earthy
6.	Pigment	: Pigmented/nonpigmented
7.	Motility (after 2 hours of incubation)	: Motile or nonmotile

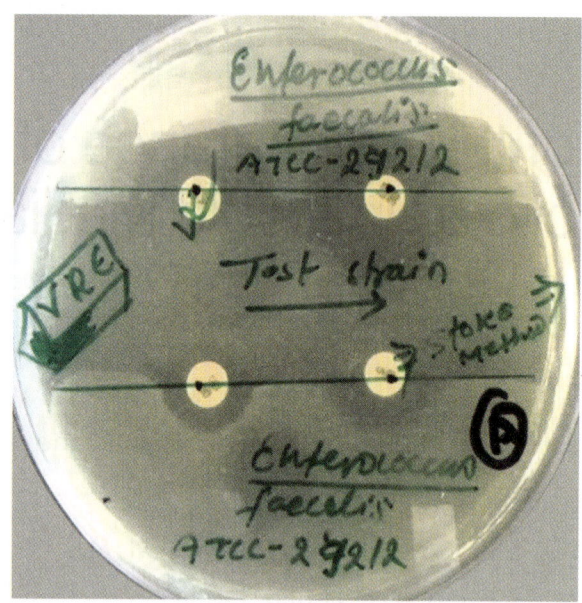

Stokes method: Test strain in centre and control strains above and below

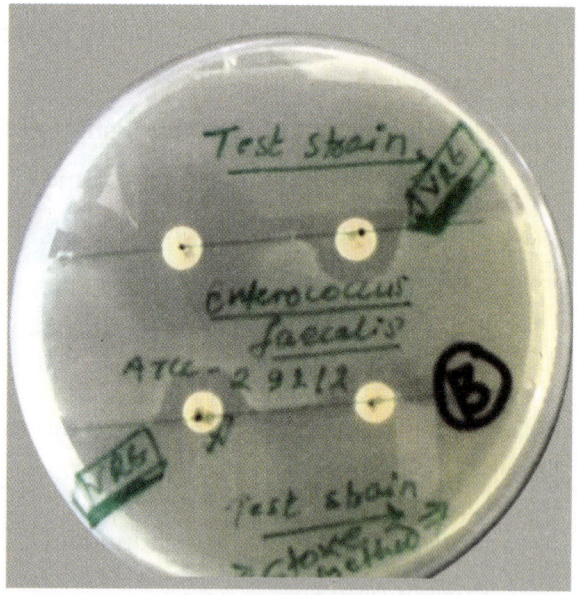

Modified Stokes method: Control strains in centre and test strains above and below. Two separate strains can be tested

Demonstration of Methods of Antimicrobial Susceptibility Testing

Aim: Antimicrobial susceptibility testing (AST) measures the ability of an antimicrobial agent to inhibit growth of microorganism *in vitro*. It is an essential step for properly treating infectious diseases and monitoring antimicrobial resistance (AMR) in various pathogens.

Minimum inhibitory concentration (MIC) is the lowest concentration of an antimicrobial that will inhibit the visible growth of a microorganism following overnight incubation.

Diffusion Method

- Media used: **Müeller Hinton agar**
- Methods used:
    - **Kirby-Bauer method** (using controls ATCC *S. aureus* 25923, *E. coli* 25922, *Pseudomonas* 27853)
    - **Stokes method** (controls NCTC *S. aureus* 6571, *E. coli* 10418, *Pseudomonas* 10662)
    - **E-test** using E-strip

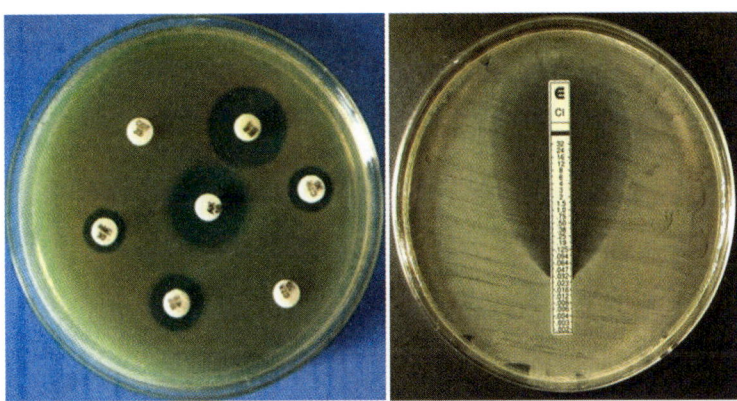

Kirby-Bauer method   E-test

Dilution Method

- Agar dilution
- Broth dilution: Macro broth dilution and micro broth dilution

Automated Systems Used

- Microscan walkaway
- Vitek 1 and 2
- Sensititre

ENTOMOLOGY

Phylum: Arthropoda
Class: Insecta, Arachnida, Crustaceae

Characteristics	Class Insecta	Class Arachnida	Class Crustaceae
Body divided into	Head Thorax Abdomen	Cephalothorax Abdomen	Cephalothorax Abdomen
Legs	3 pairs	**Ticks:** Adult—4 pairs Larvae—3 pairs **Mites:** Egg and larva—3 pairs Nymph and adult—4 pairs	5 pairs
Antenna	1 pair	Absent	2 pairs
Wings	**Absent:** Lice, flea, bug **Present:** **1 pair**—mosquito, sandfly, housefly, tsetse fly **2 pairs**—cockroach, reduviid bug	Absent	Absent
Examples	Mosquito, fly, lice, flea, bug	Ticks and mites	Cyclops, diaptomus crab, cray fish, fairy shrimps

ENTOMOLOGY

DISEASES TRANSMITTED BY CLASS INSECTA

	Mosquito-borne diseases
Anopheles	Malaria; Chittoor virus
Culex	Filariasis; Japanese encephalitis; West Nile fever; sindbis virus
Aedes	Dengue; chikungunya; yellow fever; viral hemorrhagic fever
Mansonoides	Filariasis
	Fly-borne diseases
Sandfly	Leishmaniasis; sandfly fever; bartonellosis; oriental sore
Tsetse fly (Glossina)	African trypanosomiasis (sleeping sickness)
Housefly (*Musca* spp.)	Mechanical carrier of diarrhea; dysentery; typhoid fever; trachoma; conjunctivitis; anthrax; yaws; myiasis
	Lice-borne diseases
Head louse (*P. capitis*)	Epidemic typhus; mechanical irritation, dermatitis
Body louse (*P. corporis*)	Epidemic typhus; trench fever; relapsing fever
Pubic louse (*Phthirus pubis*)	No disease India
	Flea-borne diseases
Rat flea (*Xenopsylla cheopis*)	Plague; endemic typhus; murine typhus; cestode infection due to *H. diminuta*
	Bug-borne diseases
Cone nosed bugs (reduviid bugs)	Chagas disease (American trypanosomiasis)

ENTOMOLOGY

DISEASES TRANSMITTED BY CLASS ARACHNIDA

	Ticks-borne diseases
Hard tick (ixodid tick) *Dermacentor* spp., *Rhipicephalus* spp. *Haemaphysalis, Ixodes, Amblyomma*	Relapsing fever; tularemia; babesiosis; Lyme disease; Rocky Mountain spotted fever; viral encephalitis (KFD) viral hemorrhagic fever; RSSE
Soft tick—Argasidae.	Relapsing fever, KFD
	Mite-borne diseases
Scrub mite—trombiculid	Scrub typhus
Itch mite (*Sarcoptes scabiei*)	Scabies
Dust mite	Allergy
Rat mite	Rickettsialpox

DISEASES TRANSMITTED BY CLASS CRUSTACEAE (WATER FLEA)

	Crustaceae-borne diseases
Small crustaceans (cyclops, diaptomus)	Dracunculosis, *D. latum* infection
Big crustaceans (crab, cray fish, fairy shrimps)	Transmitting the metacercariae of *P. westermani* (lung fluke)

Miscellaneous
Arthropods of Medical Importance
(Including Tables)

Aim: To study characteristic features of various insects/vectors and diseases transmitted to man.

1. *Anopheles* mosquito
2. *Aedes* mosquito
3. Mosquito larvae
4. Housefly
5. Tsetse fly
6. Sandfly
7. Cyclops
8. Hard tick
9. Soft tick
10. Rat flea
11. Itch mite
12. Louse

Characteristic Features of Adult *Anopheles* Mosquito

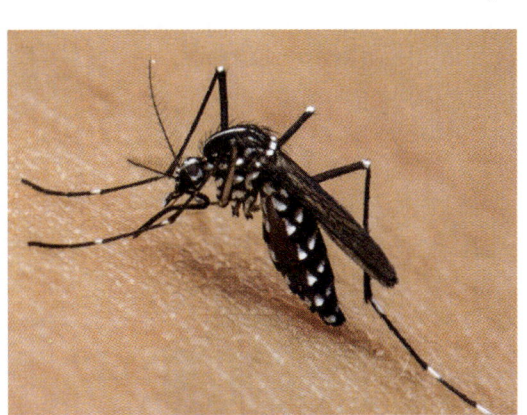

- Adult sits at an angle.
- Wings are spotted at the periphery.
- Diseases transmitted—malaria, Chittoor virus.

Adult *Anopheles* mosquito

Characteristic Features of Adult *Aedes* Mosquito

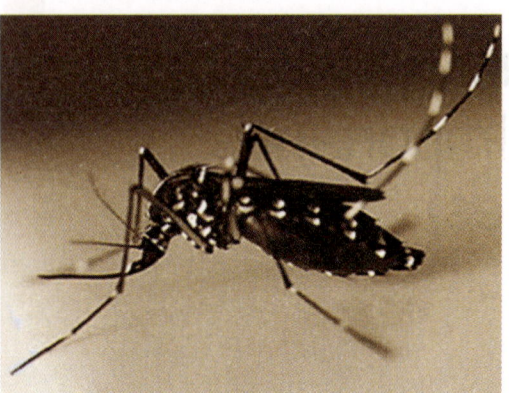

- White stripes on its black body and legs (Tiger mosquito)
- Bites during daytime
- Breeds in clean stagnant water
- Abundant during rainy season
- Diseases transmitted—chikungunya, dengue, yellow fever.

Adult *Aedes* mosquito

Mosquito Larvae

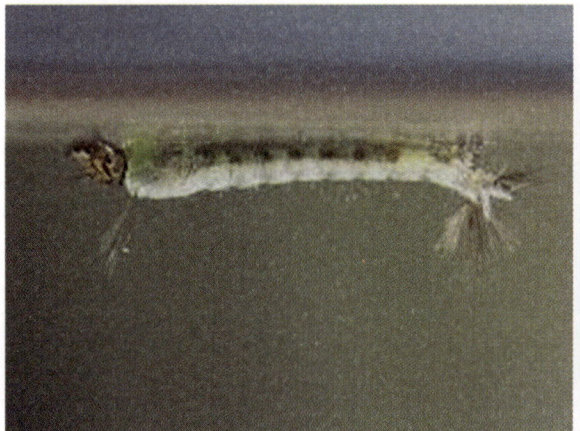

***Anophelini (Anopheles)* larva**

- Rests parallel to water surface
- No siphon tube
- Palmate hairs present on abdominal segments.

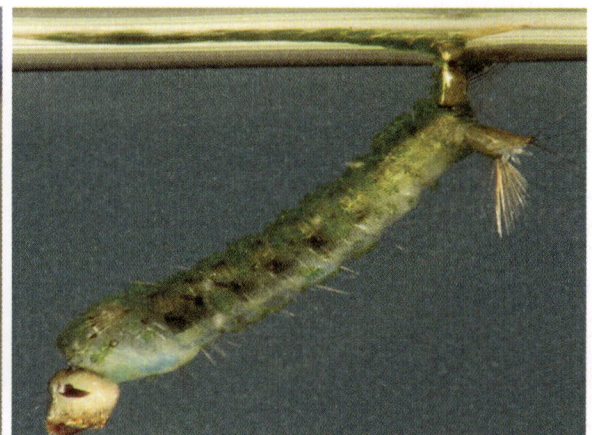

Culicine (Culex, Aedes, Mansonia) larva

- Suspended with head downwards at an angle to water surface.
- Siphon tube present
- No palmate hairs

Characteristic Features of Housefly

- A pair of antennae, short retractile proboscis, compound eye
- Thorax bears a pair of wings and three pairs of hairy legs
- Act as mechanical transmitters of diseases like enteric fever, gastroenteritis causing agents, trachoma, myiasis, etc.

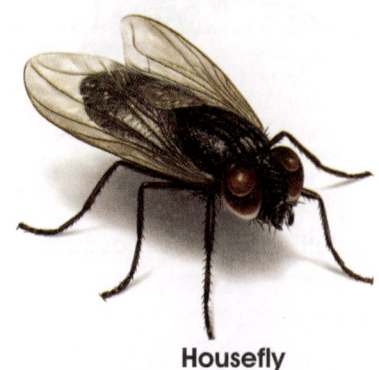

Housefly

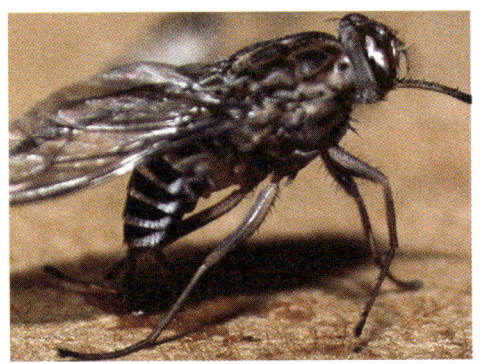

Tsetse fly

Characteristic Features of Tsetse Fly

- Yellow or dark brown—resembles housefly
- Wings when folded overlap each other like blades of scissors
- Rigid, nonretractile proboscis adapted for skin piercing
- Disease transmitted trypanosomiasis—"sleeping sickness".

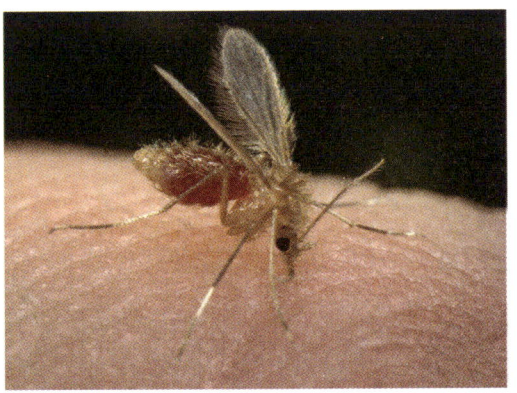

Sandfly

Characteristic Features of Sandfly

- Small insect 1.5–2 mm in length—body and wings densely haired
- Long slender and hairy antennae, palpi and proboscis
- Thorax bears a pair of wings and three pairs of legs
- Wings are upright and lanceolate, hairy—second longitudinal vein branches twice with first branching at the middle of the wing—characteristic of the genus *Phlebotomus*.
- Legs are long and slender and out of proportion to the body
- Sandflies hop and do not fly.
- Transmit leishmaniasis.

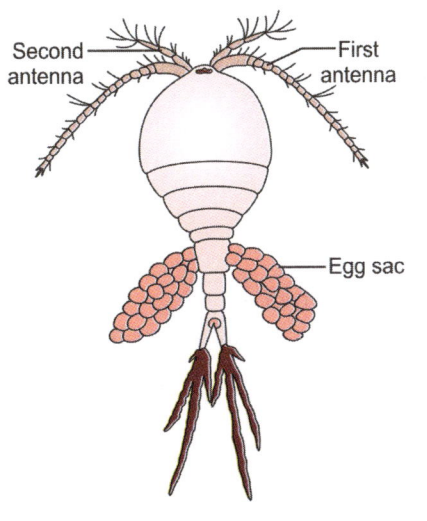

Cyclops

Characteristic Features of Cyclops

- Not more than 1 mm in length
- Pear-shaped semi-transparent body
- Forked tail
- 2 pairs of antennae
- 5 pairs of legs
- A small pigmented eye
- Transmits dracunculiasis and fish tapeworm (*Diphyllobothrium latum*) infestation

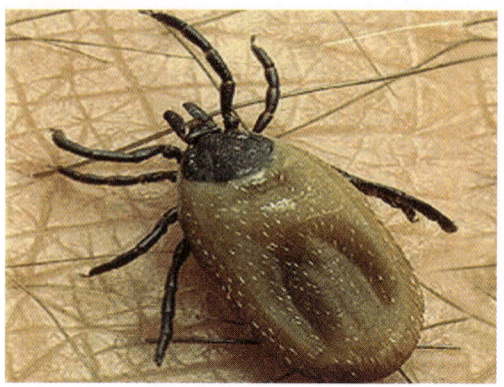

Hard tick

Characteristic Features of Hard Tick

- Scutum present—entire in males, small portion in front in females
- Head anterior
- Several hundred or thousand eggs laid at one sitting
- Cannot starve—bites day and night
- Diseases transmitted: Babesious, tularemia, tick typhus Lyme disease

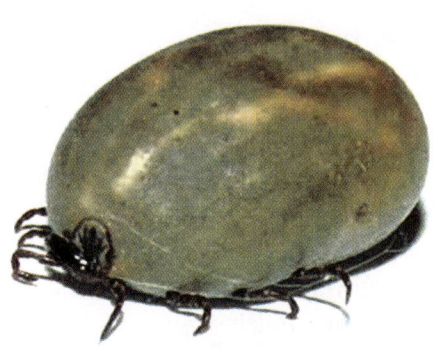

Soft tick

Characteristic Features of Soft Tick

- Scutum absent
- Head ventral—not seen from above
- Laid in batches 20–100 over a long period of time
- Can starve for a year or more
- Diseases transmitted—borreliasis, relapsing fever, Q-fever, KFD

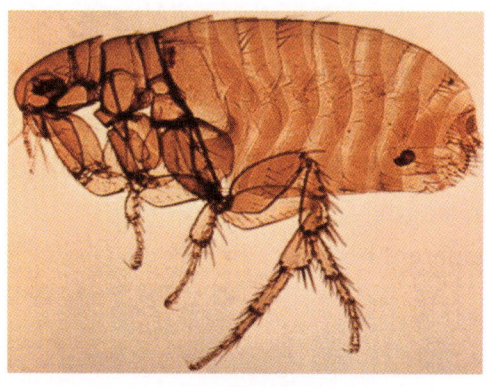

Rat flea

Characteristic Features of Rat Flea

- The insect is laterally flattened
- Conical head without a neck—piercing mouth parts project downwards and are conspicuous
- Three segmented thorax—pro-, meso- and meta-thorax—no wings
- Three pairs of strong legs
- 10 segmented abdomen—males have a coiled structure—the penis; females have a short, stumpy structure—the spermatheca
- **Cannot fly—jumps** vertically 4 inches when starved or 3 inches when fed and can jump horizontally up to 6 inches
- Diseases transmitted: Endemic typhus and bubonic plague.

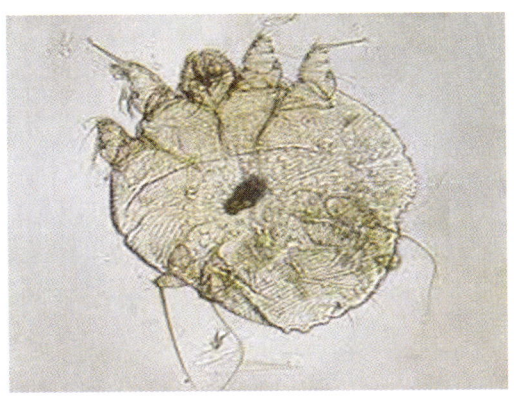

Itch mite

Characteristic Features of Itch Mite

- 0.4 mm size
- **Body:** No demarcation between cephalothorax and abdomen.
    - 2 pairs of legs in front—suckers
    - 2 pairs of legs behind—long bristle
- Male has sucker in all the legs except the 3rd pair which distinguishes it from female.
- Disease transmitted: Scabies

Characteristic Features of Louse

- Head is pointed in front, 5 jointed antennae, mouth parts adapted for sucking blood
- Thorax fused mass, square-shaped
- Strongly built three pairs of legs with claws
- 9-segmented elongated abdomen
- **Diseases transmitted:**
    - Epidemic typhus
    - Relapsing fever (epidemic)
    - Trench fever
    - Dermatitis
- **Species:**
    - Head louse—*Pediculus capitis*
    - Body louse—*Pediculus corporis*
    - Pubic or crab louse—*Phthirus pubis*

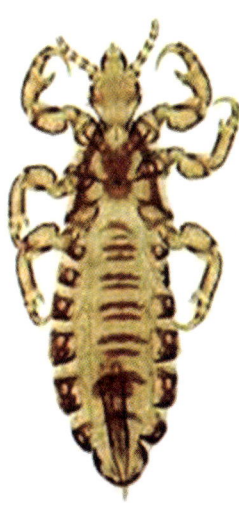

Head louse   Body louse

Demonstration of Methods for Diagnosis of Viral Infections

Aim: To study the different routes of inoculation for isolation of viruses from embryonated hen's egg and different methods for diagnosis of viruses.

Demonstration

1. Tissue culture bottle
2. Viral transport medium
3. Microtitre plate
4. Methods of inoculation of embryonated eggs
5. Hemagglutination test
6. Multinucleated giant cells of HSV
7. Negri body

Microtitre Plate

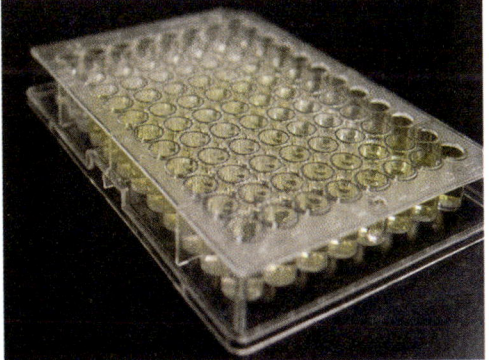

- It is a flat plate with multiple "wells" (96 wells).
- Made of polystyrene, polypropylene or polycarbonate.
- Wells have either a conical/flat/round bottom.
- Uses:
    - ELISA for diagnosis of HIV, HBV, HCV.
    - Hemagglutination test
    - Hemagglutination inhibition test
    - Complement fixation.
    - TPHA test (*Treponema pallidum* hemagglutination)

Microtitre plate

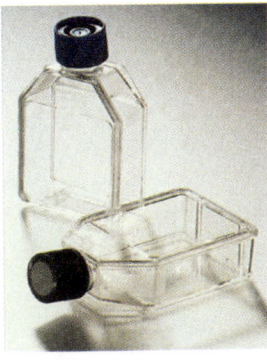

Tissue culture bottles

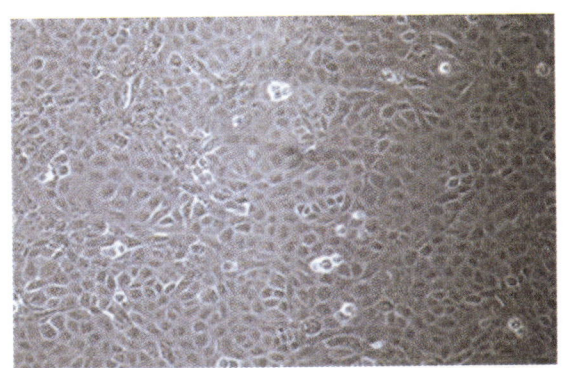

A monolayer of vero cell (vervet monkey kidney cell, continuous cell line)

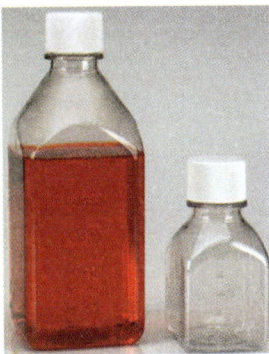

Viral transport medium (pink to red)

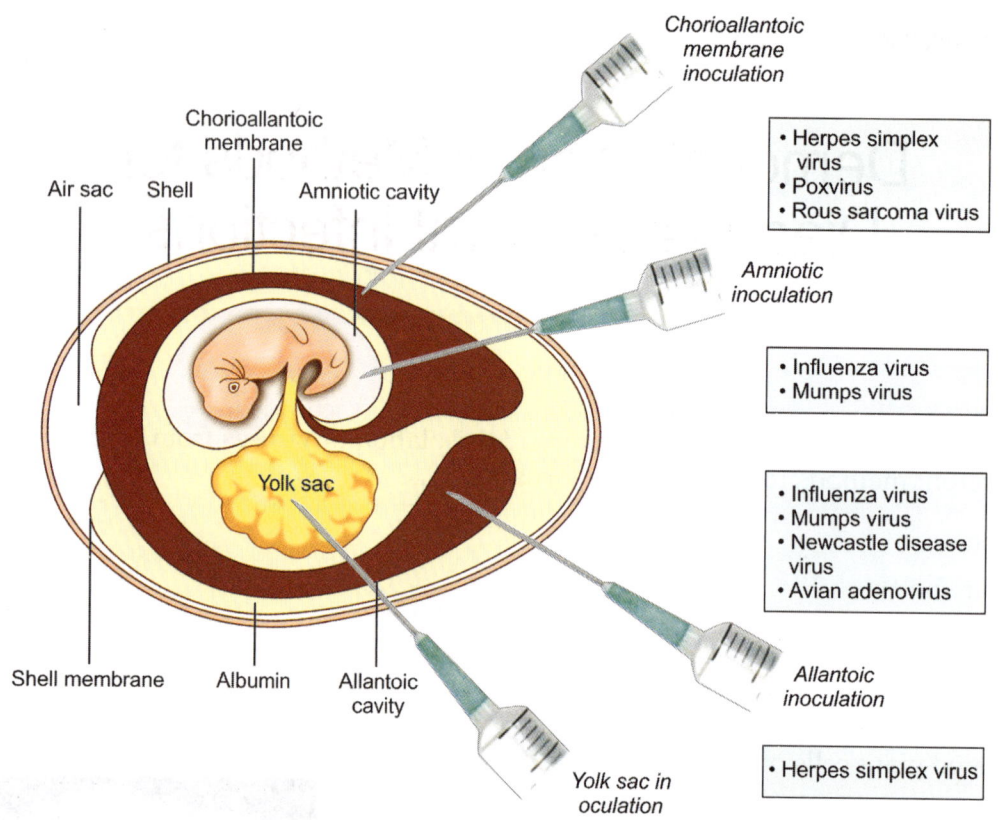

Growth of viruses in embryonated hen's egg
An embryonated chicken egg showing the different compartments in which viruses may grow.
The different routes by which viruses are inoculated into eggs are indicated.

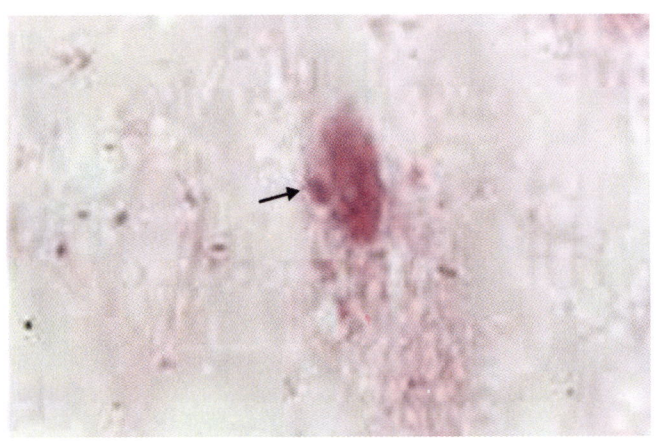

Impression smear from hippocampus of a rabid dog showing magenta colored intracellular Negri body (arrow) in a neuron. Seller's stain

Negri Body

- Specific intracytoplasmic eosinophilic inclusion body found in the cytoplasm of large neurons (1–10/cell) in rabies
- 2–20 μm, sharply defined, spherical/oval/elongated
- Cherry red to magenta colored, uniformly stained
- Larger Negri bodies contain blue staining granules/inner bodies, often arranged in concentric layers
- Part of the brain that best demonstrates Negri bodies is the Ammon horn of hippocampus
- Stain used: Seller stain
- Negri bodies are found in infection with street virus but not fixed virus
- Sensitivity of Negri bodies in rabies is 65–68%.

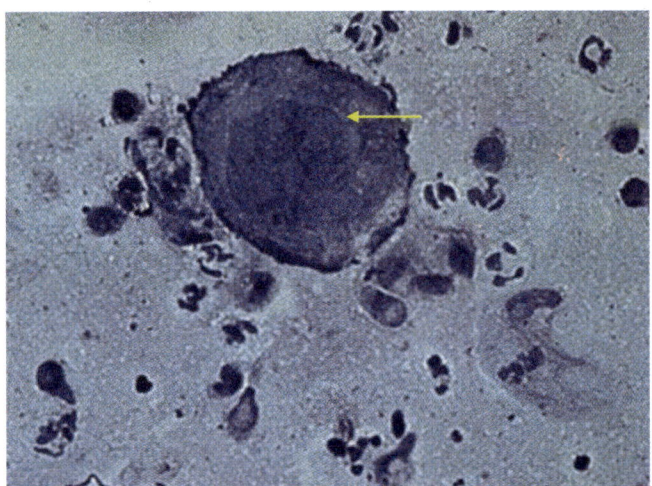

Giemsa stained Tzank smear from genital ulcer showing multinucleated giant cells of HSV-2

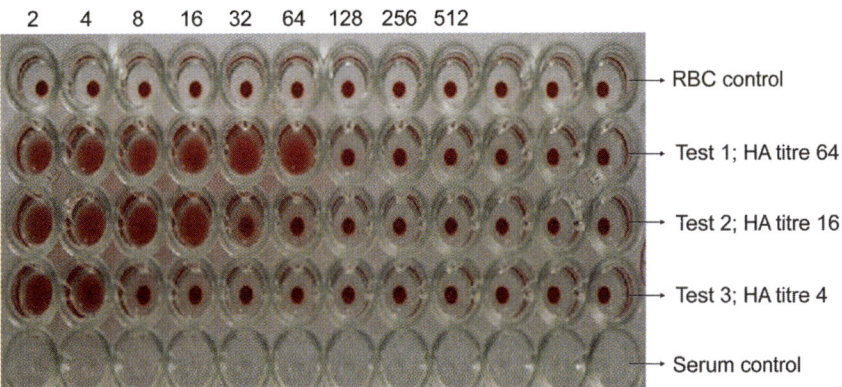

Hemagglutination test

Antigen–Antibody Reactions

IMMUNOLOGY

Antigen (Ag)–antibody (Ab) reaction (conventional)—agglutination and precipitation
Antigen–antibody reaction (newer)—ELISA, ELFA, CLIA, IFA, Western blot, rapid methods.

ANTIGEN–ANTIBODY REACTION

At the end of the session, the students shall be able to:

1. Enumerate different immunological tests available for diagnosis of infectious diseases.
2. Describe the principle, types and application of agglutination test.
3. Describe the principle, and application of precipitation test.
4. Describe the principle, application of ELISA test.
5. Describe the principle, types and application of immunofluorescence test.

PRECIPITATION REACTIONS

When a **soluble antigen** reacts with its antibody in the presence of optimal temperature, pH, electrolytes, it leads to formation of antigen–antibody complex.

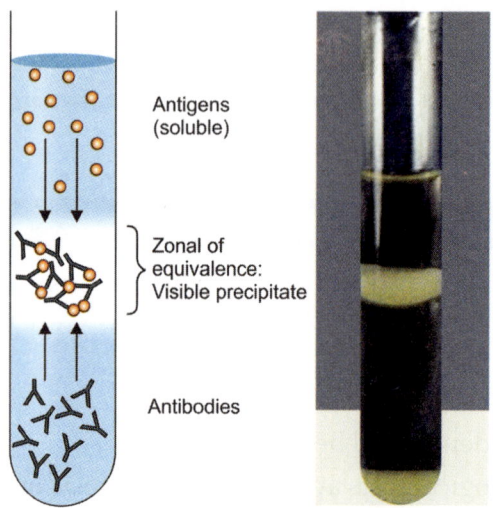

Precipitation test

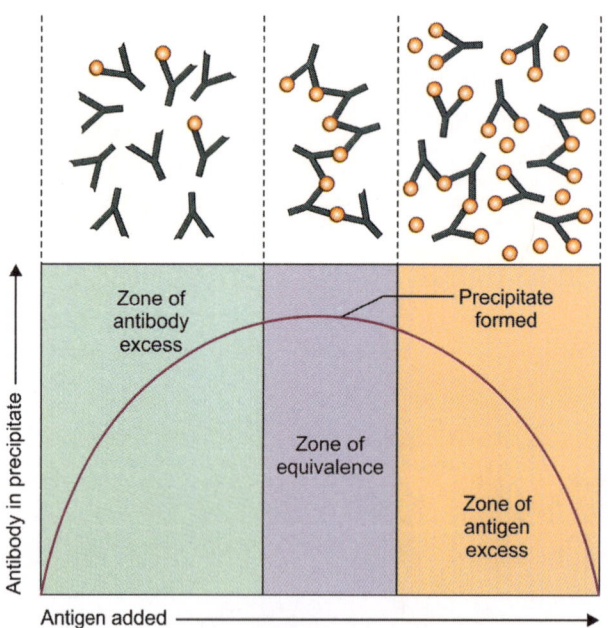

Precipitation curve

TYPES

- Immunodiffusion: On gel or agar medium insoluble precipitation bands are seen. Or in presence of electric current is known as immune electrophoresis.
- Flocculation: Insoluble floccules form in liquid medium.

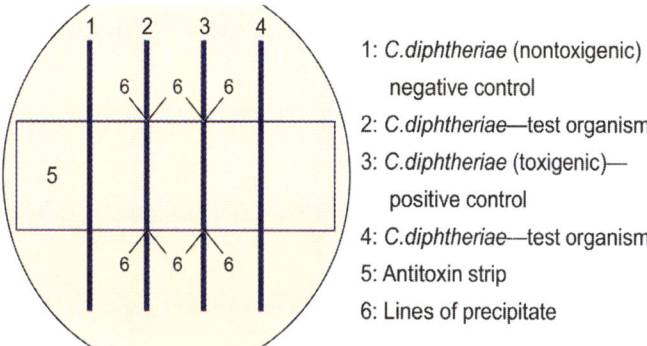

1: *C.diphtheriae* (nontoxigenic) negative control
2: *C.diphtheriae*—test organism
3: *C.diphtheriae* (toxigenic)— positive control
4: *C.diphtheriae*—test organism
5: Antitoxin strip
6: Lines of precipitate

Elek's gel precipitation test

Slide Flocculation Test

Procedure: A drop of antigen is mixed with a drop of patients serum containing antibody on a slide, the precipitate formed remain suspended as floccules.

Venereal Disease Research Laboratory (VDRL test).

AGGLUTINATION REACTION

When a **particulate or insoluble antigen** is mixed with its antibody in the presence of electrolytes at a suitable temperature and pH, the particles are agglutinated.

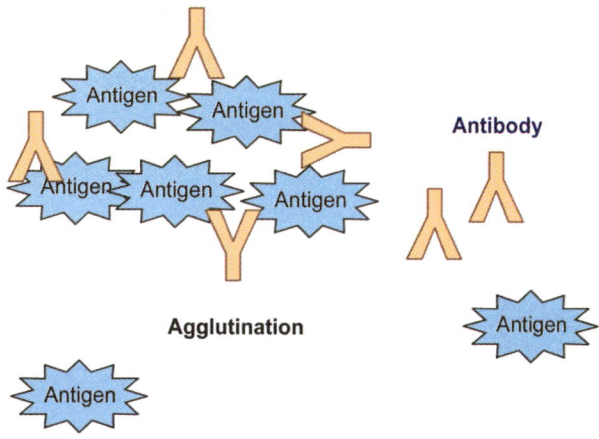

- **Direct agglutination reaction** (slide or tube agglutination reaction)

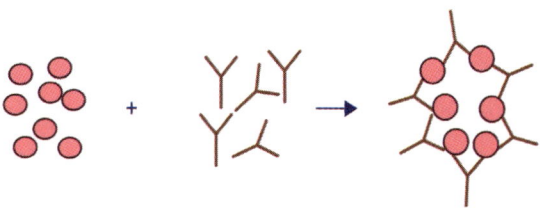

Direct agglutination reaction

- **Indirect or passive agglutination test:** For antibody detection
  a. Indirect haemagglutination assay reaction (IHA)

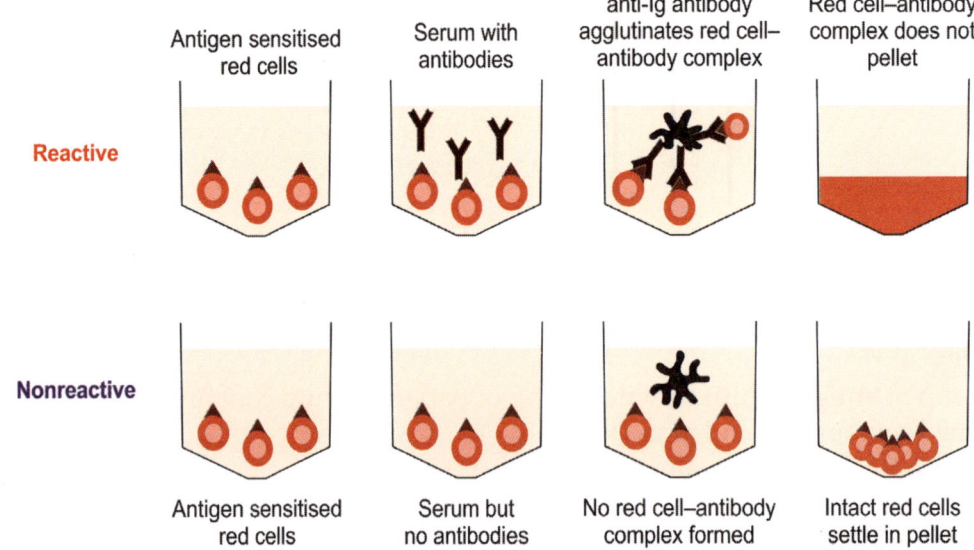

Indirect haemagglutination

b. Latex agglutination test/reaction (LAT); for antibody

  - **Reverse passive agglutination test:** For antigen detection

    (a) Reverse passive haemagglutination assay/test (RPHA): HBsAg detection
    (b) Latex agglutination test, e.g. CRP, Cryptococcus antigen

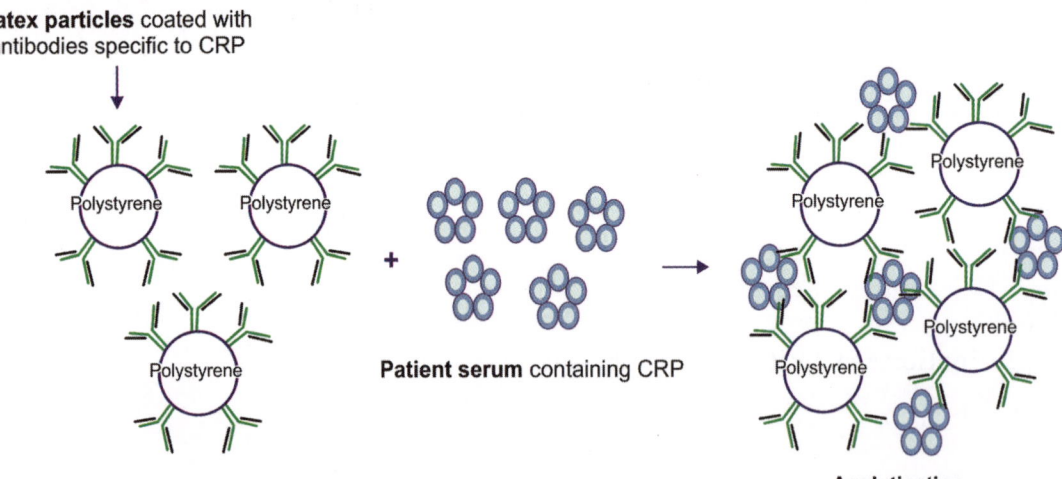

c. **Conglutination test:** *Staphylococcus aureus* detection

  - **Haemagglutination Test**

    (a) **Direct haemagglutination test,** e.g. Paul Bunnel test, blood group

COMPLEMENT FIXATION TEST

Detection of antibodies to Chlamydia, Mycoplasma, arboviral infections.

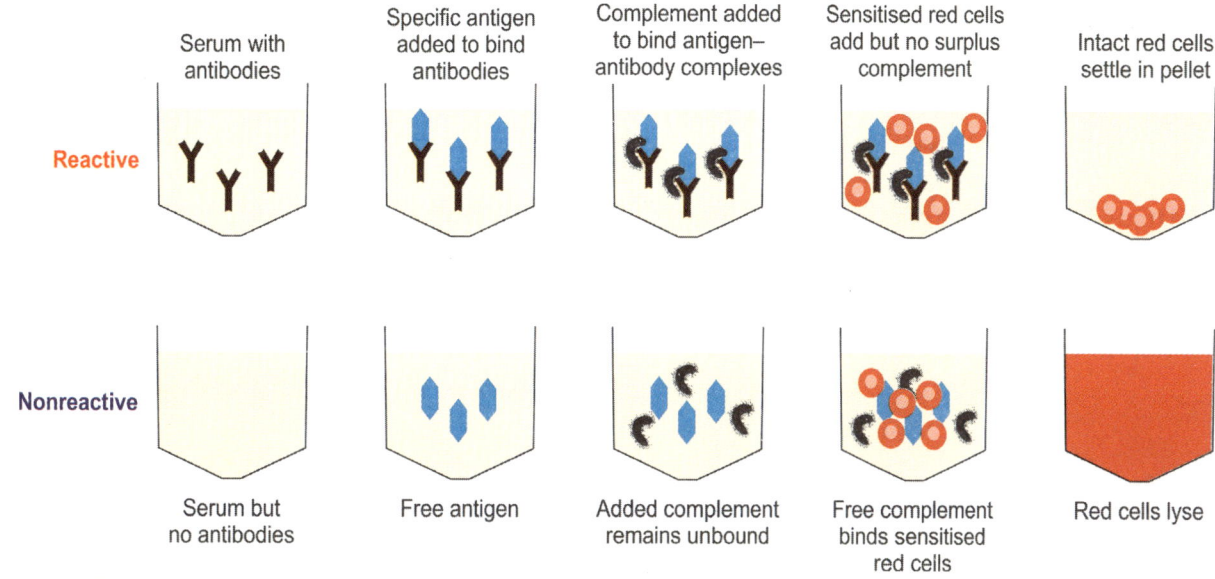

| Reactive | Serum with antibodies | Specific antigen added to bind antibodies | Complement added to bind antigen–antibody complexes | Sensitised red cells add but no surplus complement | Intact red cells settle in pellet |

| Nonreactive | Serum but no antibodies | Free antigen | Added complement remains unbound | Free complement binds sensitised red cells | Red cells lyse |

Complement fixation test

NEUTRALIZATION TEST

a. Viral neutralization test

b. Plaque inhibition test

c. Toxin-antitoxin neutralization test (ASO, Schick test, Naglers reaction)

d. Haemagglutination inhibition (HAI) test: Influenza

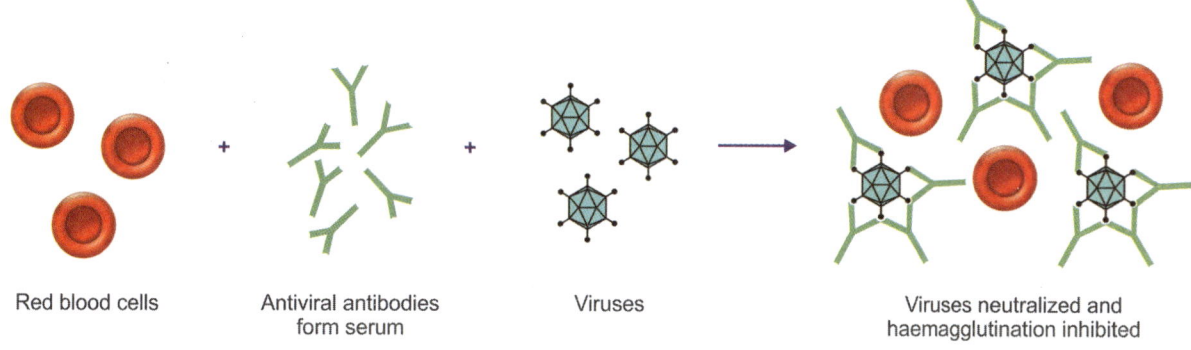

| Red blood cells | Antiviral antibodies form serum | Viruses | Viruses neutralized and haemagglutination inhibited |

NEWER TECHNIQUES

Enzyme-linked Immunosorbent Assay

It detects either the antigen or the antibody in the specimen by using enzyme–substrate–sorbent–chromogen system for detection.

Principle of ELISA: An adsorbing material is used (polystyrene plate) to adsorb antigen or antibody. Then enzyme is used to label these components. It reacts with the substrate which activates the chromogen to produce color (e.g. horseradish peroxidase).

Substrate chromogen system is added to complete the reaction. The color change is detected by spectrophotometry.

Ag + Ab complex–enzyme–substrate–activates chromogen–color–detected by ELISA reader.

TYPES OF ELISA

- **Direct ELISA:** In a direct ELISA, an antigen or sample is immobilized directly on the plate and a conjugated detection antibody binds to the target protein. Substrate is then added, producing a signal that is proportional to the amount of analyte in the sample. Since only one antibody is used in a direct ELISA, they are less specific than a sandwich ELISA.

  When to use: Assessing antibody affinity and specificity. Investigating blocking/inhibitory interactions.

  Advantages: Fast and simple protocol

  Disadvantages: Less specific since you are only using 1 antibody.

  Potential for high background if all proteins from a sample are immobilized in well.

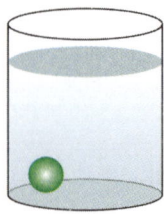 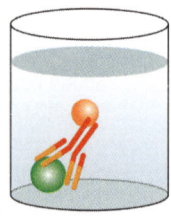 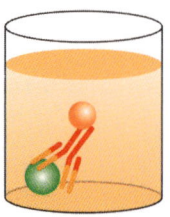

- **Indirect ELISA:** An indirect ELISA is similar to a direct ELISA in that an antigen is immobilized on a plate, but it includes an additional amplification detection step. First, an unconjugated primary detection antibody is added and binds to the specific antigen. A conjugated secondary antibody directed against the host species of the primary antibody is then added. Substrate then produces a signal proportional to the amount of antigen bound in the well.

  When to Use: Measuring endogenous antibodies.

  Advantages: Amplification using a secondary antibody.

  Disadvantages: Potential for cross-reactivity caused by secondary antibody.

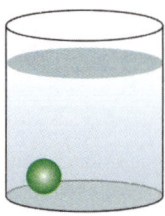 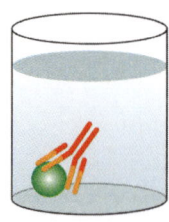 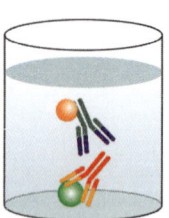 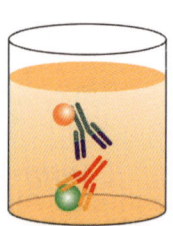

- **Sandwich ELISA:** Sandwich ELISAs are the most common type of ELISA. Two specific antibodies are used to sandwich the antigen, commonly referred to as matched antibody pairs. Capture antibody is coated on a microplate, sample is added, and the protein of interest binds and is immobilized on the plate. A conjugated-detection antibody is then added and binds to an additional epitope on the target protein. Substrate is added and produces a signal that is proportional to the amount of analyte present in the sample. Sandwich ELISAs are highly specific, since two antibodies are required to bind to the protein of interest.

  When to Use: Determining analyte concentration in a biological sample.

  Advantages: Highest specificity and sensitivity. Compatible with complex sample matrices.

Disadvantages: Longer protocol. Challenging to develop.

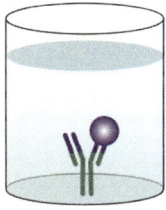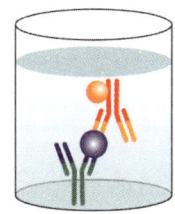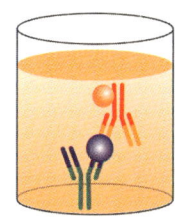

- **MAC ELISA**

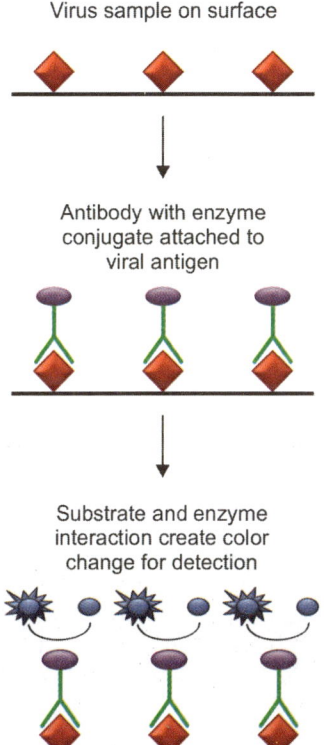

Virus sample on surface

Antibody with enzyme
conjugate attached to
viral antigen

Substrate and enzyme
interaction create color
change for detection

- **Competitive ELISA**

Competitive ELISAs are commonly used for small molecules, when the protein of interest is too small to efficiently sandwich with two antibodies. Similar to a sandwich ELISA, a capture antibody is coated on a microplate. Instead of using a conjugated detection antibody, a conjugated antigen is used to complete for binding with the antigen present in the sample. The more antigen present in the sample, the less conjugated antigen will bind to the capture antibody. Substrate is added and the signal produced is inversely proportional to the amount of protein present in the sample.

When to Use: Determining concentrations of a small molecules and hormones.

Advantages: Ability to quantitate small molecules.

Disadvantages: Less specific since you are only using 1 antibody. Requires a conjugated antigen.

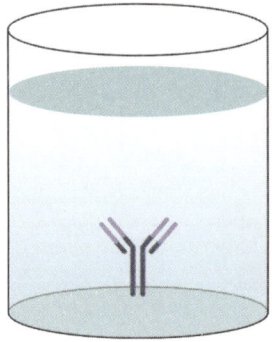
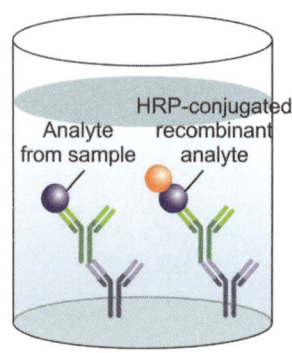
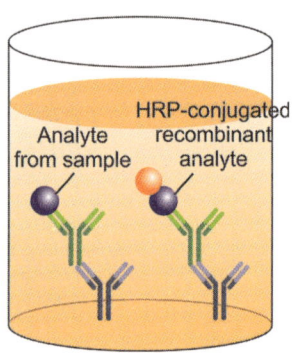

IMMUNOFLUORESCENCE ASSAY (IFA)

Principle: Specific Ab binds to the Ag of interest. Fluorescent dyes are coupled to these Ag–Ab complexes in order to visualize the Ag of interest using immunofluorescent microscope.

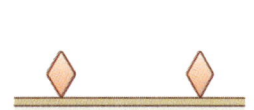
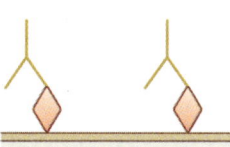
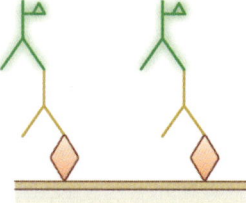

Antigen is fixed to a surface

Patient serum is added; if antibodies are present, they bind to the antigen

Secondary antibody (with fluorescent label) is added; if patient antibodies are present, the secondary antibody binds to the patient antibodies

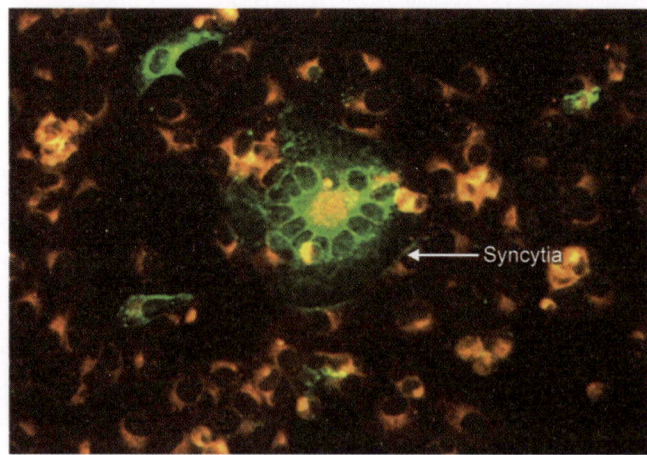

CHEMILUMINESCENCE-LINKED IMMUNOASSAY (CLIA)

Principle: In the presence of complimentary Ag and Ab, the paratope of the Ab binds to the epitope of the Ag to form Ag–Ab complex which is estimated using labeled Ab, chemiluminescent substrates and H_2O_2 as enhancer resulting in generation of light whose intensity is directly proportional to amount of labeled immune complex, e.g. detection of SARS-CoV-2 Ab.

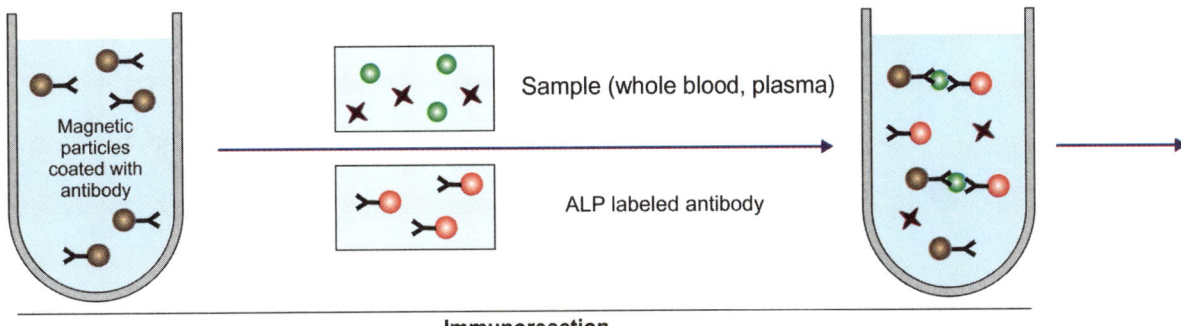

Magnetic particles coated with antibody

Sample (whole blood, plasma)

ALP labeled antibody

Immunoreaction

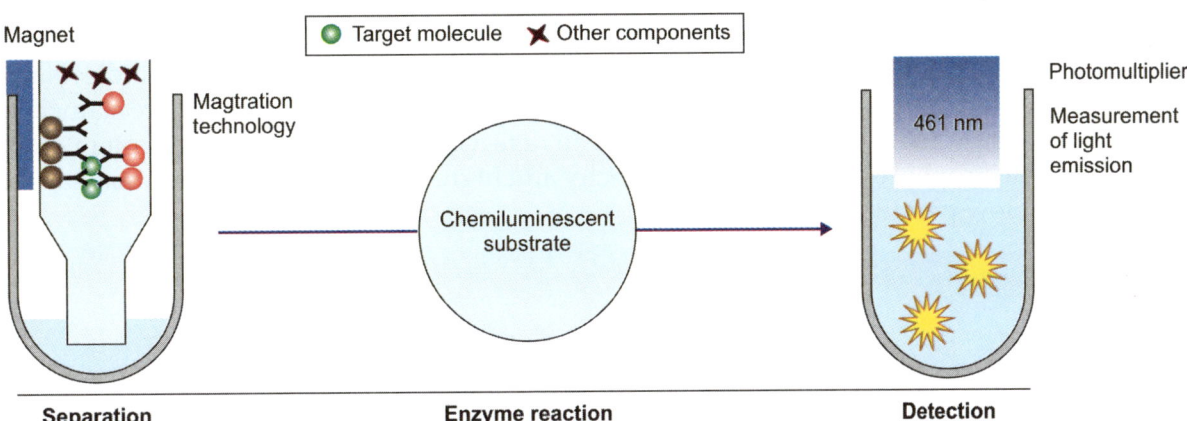

Magnet

○ Target molecule ✗ Other components

Magtration technology

Chemiluminescent substrate

Photomultiplier

461 nm

Measurement of light emission

Separation   **Enzyme reaction**   **Detection**

WESTERN BLOT

Also called protein immunoblotting used to detect specific proteins in a given sample.

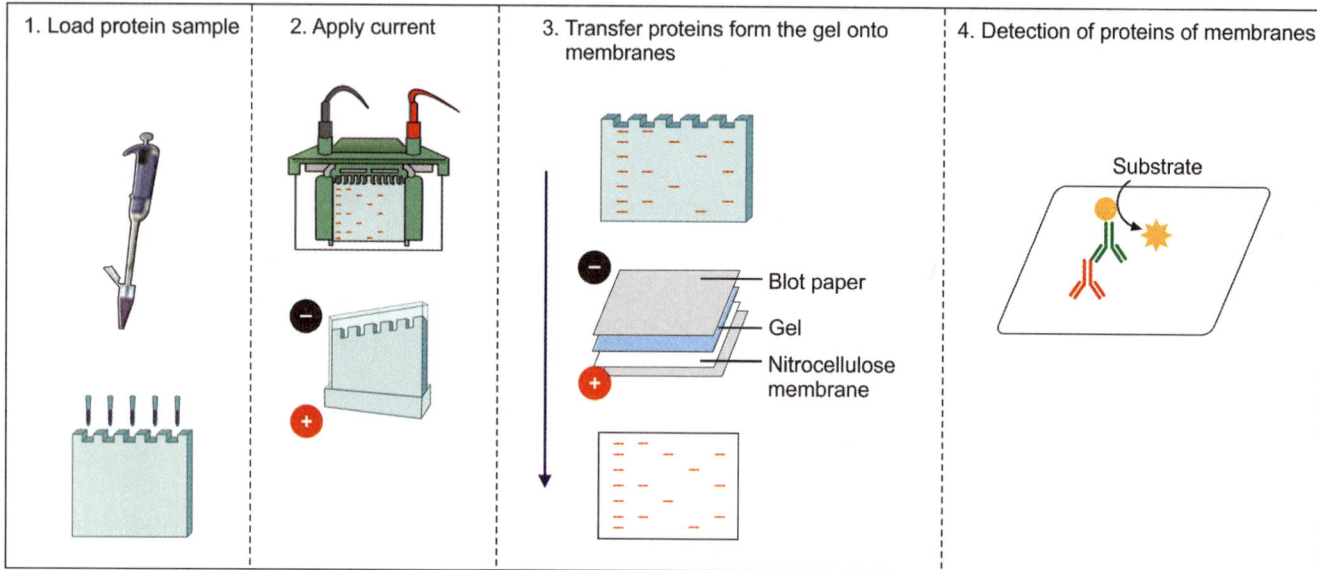

| 1. Load protein sample | 2. Apply current | 3. Transfer proteins form the gel onto membranes | 4. Detection of proteins of membranes |

Principle: Uses SDS-PAGE to separate various proteins in a sample based on their molecular weight which are then blotted or transferred onto a matrix (generally NC paper) where they are stained with Ab specific to the target protein by immunoassay. WB can detect as low as 1 ng of target protein due to high resolution of gel electrophoresis and strong specificity and high sensitivity of the immunoassay, e.g. p-24 Ag of HIV in window period.

Section
2

Perform and Identify the Different Causative Agents of Infectious Diseases by Microscopy

Demonstration of Formol-ether Concentration Method for Stool Examination

Reagents Required

1. 10% formal saline
2. Diethyl ether
3. Sieve with holes with size of 40 meshes to an inch.
4. Stool for sedimentation

Procedure

- Take stool (~1 gm, i.e. pea sized) in 10 ml distilled water in a conical bottom test tube or centrifuge tube.
- Fix the stopper on the tube and mix thoroughly by shaking for 20 seconds.
- Pass the contents through sieve → centrifuge at 2000 rpm for 1–2 minutes. Decant and discard the supernatant. Final amount of 1.0 to 1.5 ml of sediment should be present.
- Re-suspend the sediment in fresh saline → centrifuge and decant as earlier.
- Add 9.0 ml of 10% formal saline to the sediment and mix thoroughly and add 3.0 ml of ether. Stopper the tube and shake vigorously for 30 seconds.

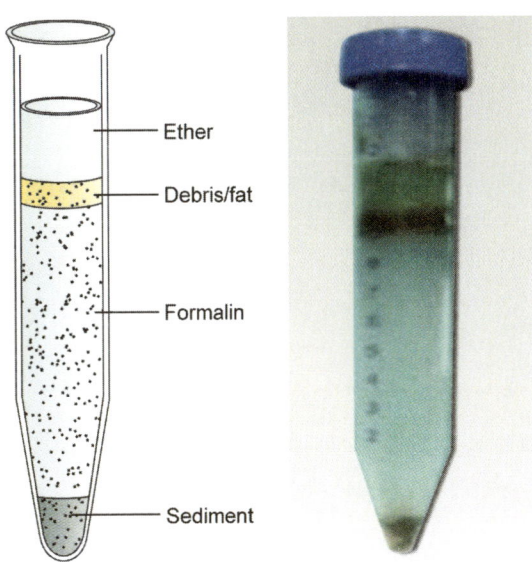

Four layers after formol-ether concentration of stool

- Centrifuge at 3000 rpm for 15 minutes. The liquid column is separated into the following four layers:
  - I. Layer of ether
  - II. Plug of debris
  - III. Layer of formalin
  - IV. Sediment
- Free the plug of debris from the sides of the tube with an application of stick and carefully decant and discard the top three layers. Use a cotton swab to clean debris from the wall of the tube.
- With a pipette, mix the remaining sediment with the small amount of fluid that drains back from the sides of the tube and prepare iodine and unstained mounts for microscopic examination.
- If examination of the specimen is delayed, add 1 or 2 ml of 10% formalin to the sediment and stopper the tube, formalized sediment may be kept for some time if dried. Remove the excess formalin before marking mounts.

Normal stool sample as observed under the microscope

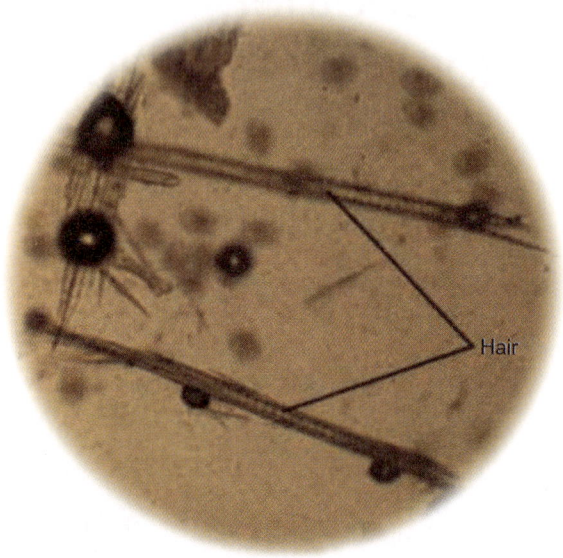

1. Plant hair

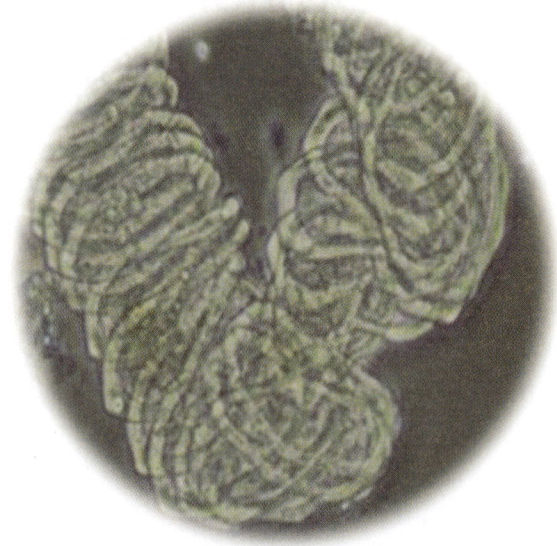

2. Vegetable spiral

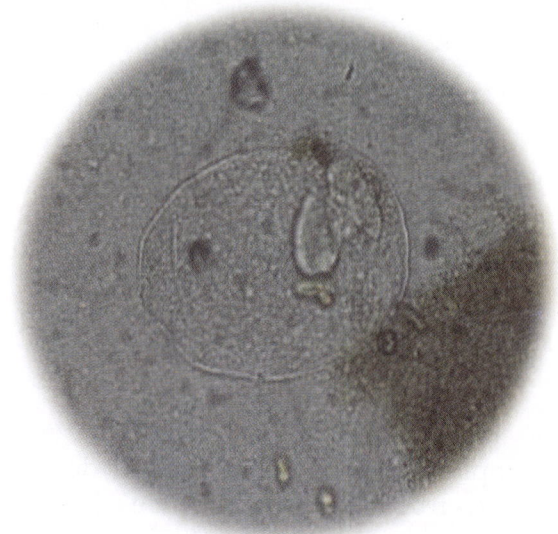

3. Vegetable cell

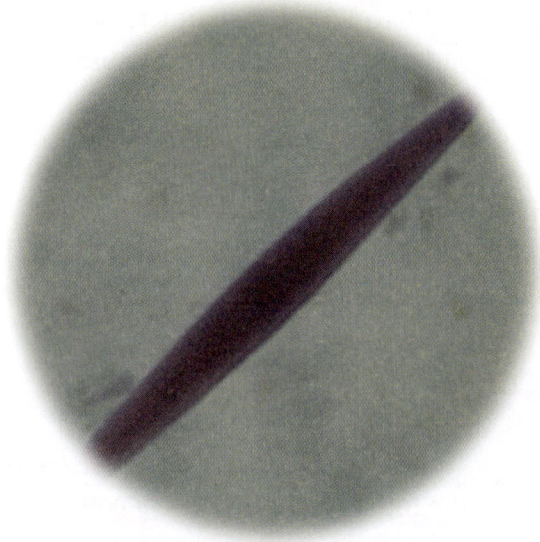

4. Abnormally seen Charcot-Leyden crystals

Demonstration of Normal Stool Findings

The following structures are commonly seen as nonpathogenic findings in a stool preparation.

1. Plant hair
- It has nondescript internal structure
- There is no head or tail region
- May resemble helminth larvae in size and shape (but no diagnostic structures).

2. Vegetable spiral
- They have a ladder-like appearance
- Often mistaken with helminth larvae (but they do not have a head or tail region).

3. Vegetable cell
- Round to oval
- Measure up to 150 μm
- Thick cell wall
- Can be confused with helminth egg (interior unorganized).

4. Abnormally seen Charcot-Leyden crystals
- These crystals are diamond-shaped
- They are eosinophilic breakdown products
- They may be found in sputum also
- Too many in quantity imply some parasitic infection.

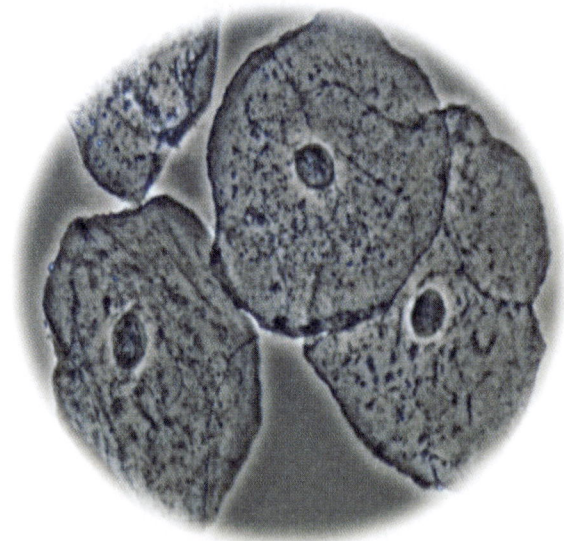

5. Epithelial cells

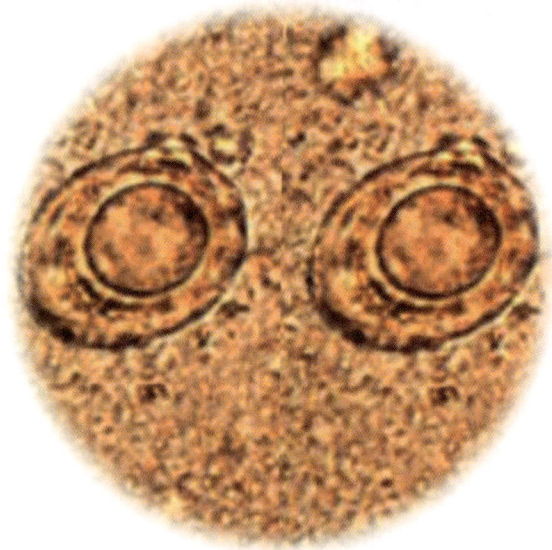

6. Pollen grains

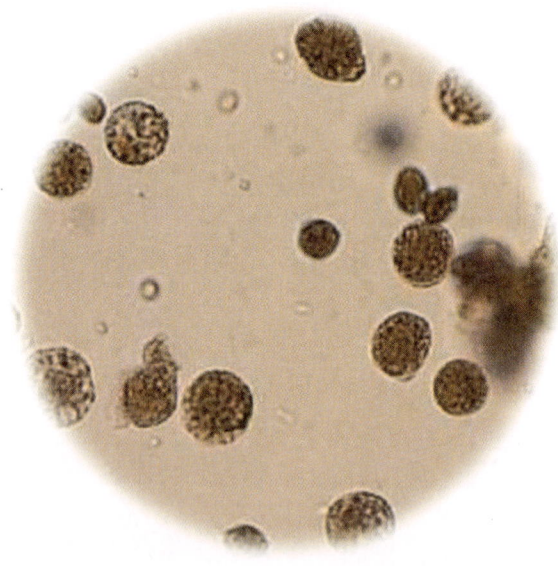

7. Abnormally seen WBCs/pus cells

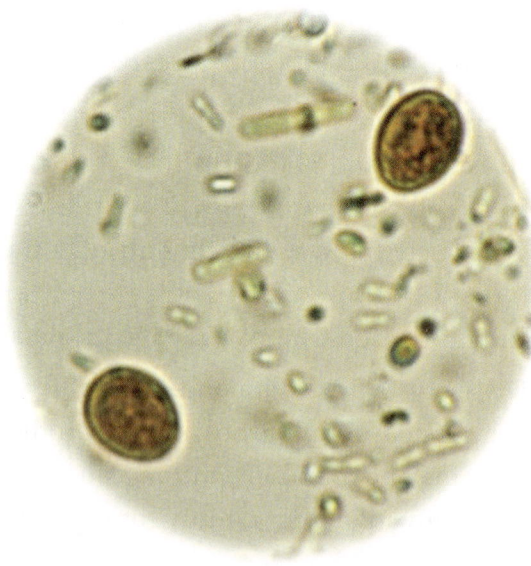

8. Yeast cells

5. Epithelial cells
- Single nucleus distinct cell wall
- Resembles amoebic trophozoite

6. Pollen grains
- Round to symmetrically lobed
- 12–20 micrometer in size
- Thick walled
- Resembling egg of *Taenia* spp. (but smaller with no notable interior structure).

7. Abnormally seen WBCs/pus cells
- Size—15 μm
- Have 2–4 lobed nucleus connected by chromatin bands
- Can be mistaken with nucleus of *E. histolytica*
- Mononuclear WBC ranges from 28 to 62 μm
- Closely resemble trophozoite of *E. histolytica*
- Degenerated WBCs are pus cells which when present in large numbers imply an invasive diarrhea.

8. Yeast cells
- Oval structures
- Confused with cysts of *Entamoeba hartmanni, E. nana* but no definite internal structures are seen.

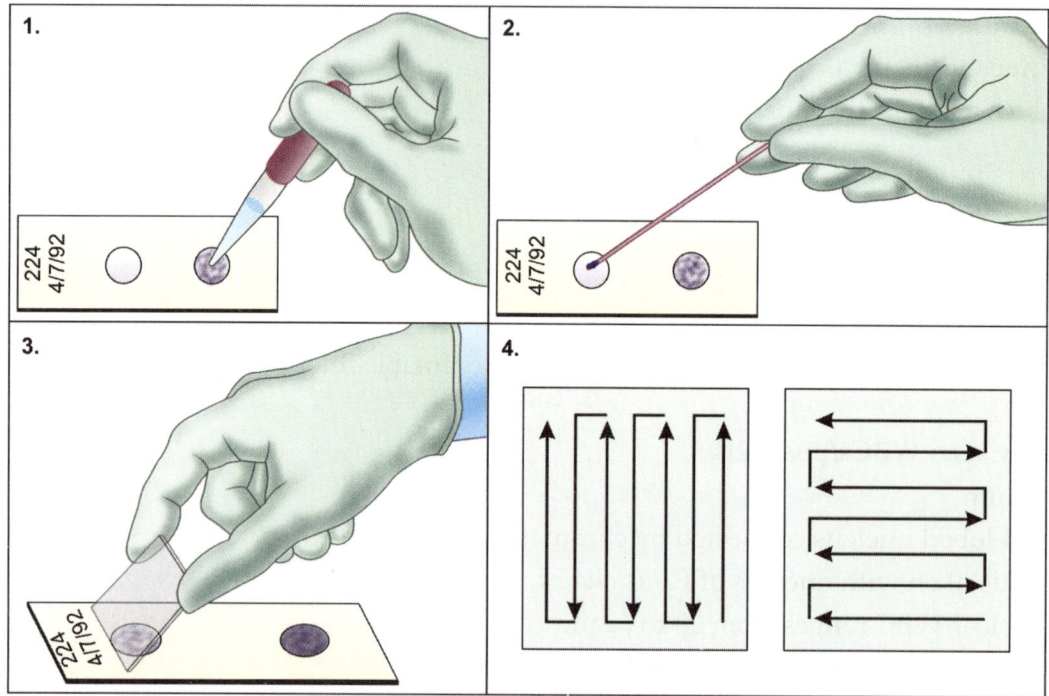

Saline and iodine mount preparation of stool on same slide

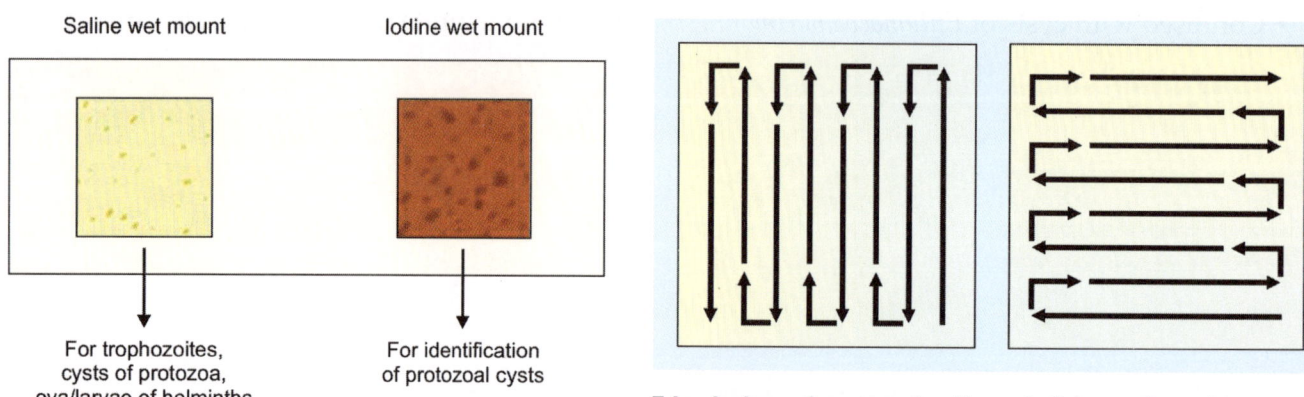

Saline wet mount

Iodine wet mount

For trophozoites,
cysts of protozoa,
ova/larvae of helminths

For identification
of protozoal cysts

Z technique for examination of slide under microscope

Preparation of Saline and Iodine Wet Mount of Stool Sample

Aim: To prepare saline and iodine wet mount of stool sample for diagnosis of ova/cysts.

Materials Required

- Clean glass slide
- Coverslip
- Stool sample
- Clean stick
- Normal saline (NS)
- Lugol's iodine
- Light microscope

Procedure

1. Take a clean slide
2. Put a drop of normal saline on one side of glass slide and of Lugol's iodine on other side.
3. With the help of separate stick, mix the stool sample in both.
4. Put the coverslip over both, drop by making an angle of 45° with slide so that bubble formation is prevented.
5. Focus the slide of normal saline under the low power objective (10X) of a light microscope so that one can see the whole area in low power.
6. An abnormal content or cyst is then focused at high power objective (40X) of a light microscope.
7. After this, iodine slide is focused at low power such that about one-third of slide is focused.
8. Confirm under high power objective.
9. The slides are scanned in a zig-zag (Z) manner.
10. Observe and note your finding first under low power objective (10X) followed by high power objective (40X) of a light microscope.

Note

i. In normal saline, one can appreciate motile trophozoites and bile-stained structures.
ii. In iodine, internal structures especially nucleus is well appreciated but one cannot see motile trophozoites as iodine inhibits motility.

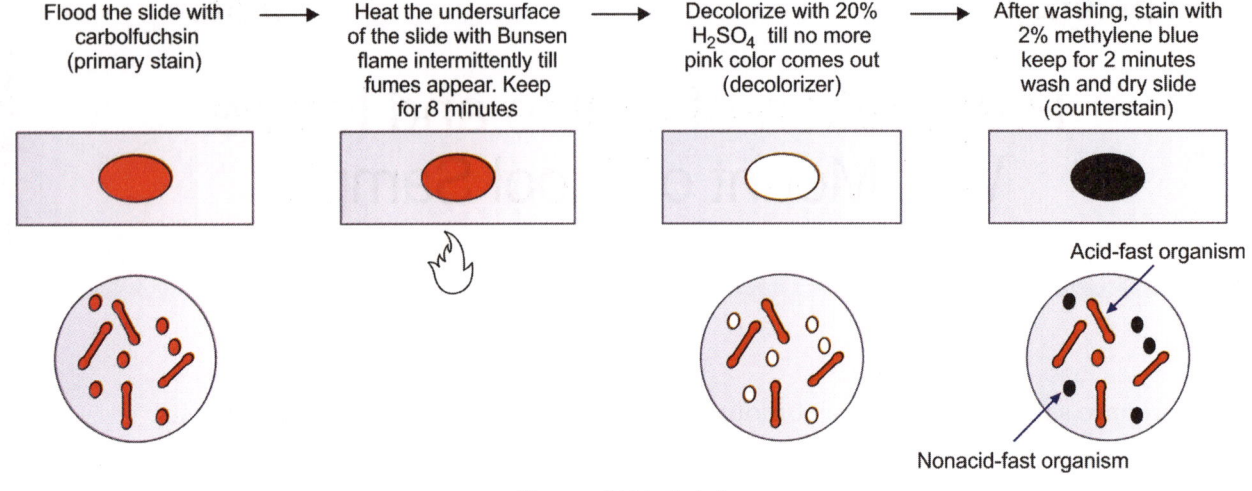

Flood the slide with carbolfuchsin (primary stain) → Heat the undersurface of the slide with Bunsen flame intermittently till fumes appear. Keep for 8 minutes → Decolorize with 20% H_2SO_4 till no more pink color comes out (decolorizer) → After washing, stain with 2% methylene blue keep for 2 minutes wash and dry slide (counterstain)

Acid-fast organism

Nonacid-fast organism

Steps of ZN stainig

Ziehl-Neelsen (ZN) Staining

Principle: Organisms such as mycobacteria are extremely difficult to stain by ordinary methods like Gram stain because of the high lipid content of their cell wall. The differential staining techniques Ziehl-Neelsen stain uses the phenolic compound carbolfuchsin which is strongly basic to bind to the mycolic acid to stain the cell wall of *Mycobacterium* species. Application of heat helps further penetration through lipoidal wall and enters into cytoplasm. Then the smear is decolorized with strong mineral acid. The ability of the bacteria to resist decolorization with acid confers acid-fastness to the bacterium. Only decolorized cells absorb the counterstain methylene blue and take its color and appear blue while acid-fast cells retain the red color of the primary stain.

Constituent of Ziehl-Neelsen Stain

- Primary stain—carbolfuchsin 0.3% (basic fuchsin + phenol + 95% alcohol)
- Decolorizer—20% H_2SO_4 or 3% acid (HCl)—alcohol can also be used
- Counterstain—2% methylene blue

Procedure

1. Heat fix the provided slide and keep on slide rack.

2. Flood slide with 0.3% carbolfuchsin and heat the undersurface of the slide with Bunsen burner flame only till fumes appear then remove heat. Do this for 8 minutes intermittently

3. Drain the slide. Do not wash.

4. Decolorize with 20% H_2SO_4 till no more pink color comes out.

5. Drain the slide and wash gently with tap water.

6. Counterstain with 2% methylene blue.

7. Wash gently with tap water and then dry.

8. Observe under 100X oil immersion objective.

Observation: Red colored bacilli with beaded appearance seen against a blue background.

Report: Acid-fast bacilli seen.

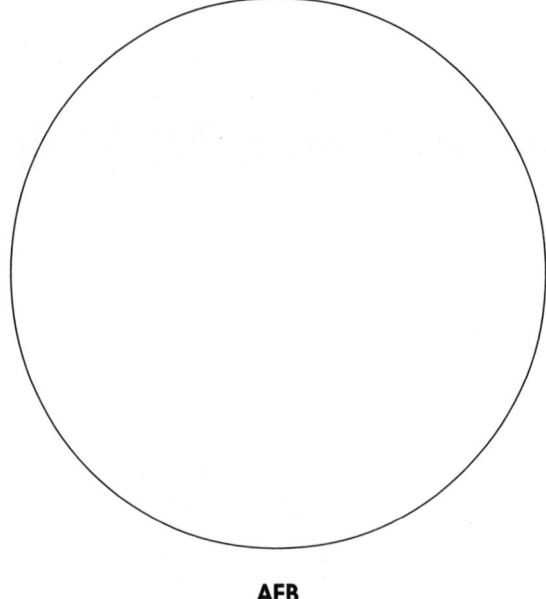

AFB

ZN Smear Evaluation and AFB Report as per RNTCP Guidelines

Grading of Slides in AFB Microscopy

Examination	Result	Grading	No. of fields to be examined
More than 10 AFB per/oil immersion fields (OIF)	Positive	3+	20
1–10 AFB/oil immersion fields	Positive	2+	50
10–99 AFB/100 oil immersion fields	Positive	1+	100
1–9 AFB/100 oil immersion fields	Positive	Scanty (record exact number seen)	100
No AFB/100 oil immersion fields	Negative	–	100

Albert Staining

Principle of Albert Staining

Albert stain is basically made up of two stains that are **toluidine blue** and **malachite green**. Its application aims at identifying bacteria that contain special structures known as metachromatic granules. Albert staining solution A acts as the staining solution while Albert solution B acts as the mordant, i.e. an ion element that binds and holds a chemical dye, to make it stuck on the micro-organism.

The bacterial cell of *Corynebacterium diphtheriae* has volutin granules in their cytoplasm which are highly acidic while the cytoplasm in neutral. Albert satin A have two dyes **toluidine blue** and **malachite green** both of which are basic dyes with high affinity for neutral tissue components like cytoplasm and the pH of Albert A is adjusted to 2.8 by using glacial acetic acid, which is acidic for cytoplasm (as it is neutral) but basic for volutin granules (as the pH of volutin granules are high acidic). Therefore, when Albert stain A applied to the cell the volutin granules stain by toluidine blue while cytoplasm stain green by malachite green. Due to the metachromatic property of volutin granules when stained with toluidine blue dye they appear red in color, but when Albert B is applied due to the effect of iodine the metachromatic property is not observed and granules appear blue black in color.

Constituent of Albert Stain

Albert A
- Toluidine blue
- Malachite green
- Glacial acetic acid
- Alcohol (95% ethanol)
- Distilled water

Albert B
- Iodine
- Potassium iodide (KI)
- Distilled water

Procedure of Albert Staining

1. Heat fix the provided slide
2. Flood slide with Albert A (through filter paper) for 5 min.
3. Drain the slide. Do not wash.
4. Flood slide with Albert B for 4 min.
5. Drain the slide and wash gently with tap water and then dry.
6. Observe under 100X oil immersion objective.

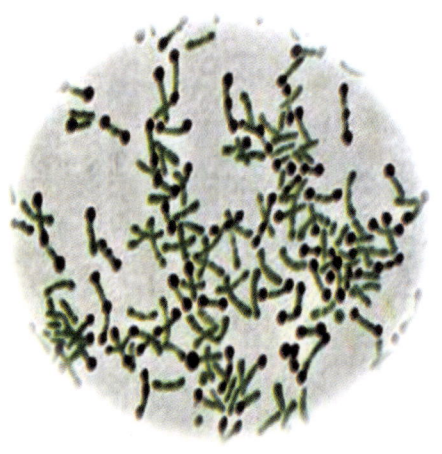

Observation: Green-colored bacilli seen with bluish black metachromatic granules at the poles. The bacilli are arranged in Chinese letter or cuneiform pattern, i.e. V- or L-shaped.

Report: Microorganisms morphologically resembling *Corynebacterium diphtheriae* are seen.

To Stain a Smear by Gram Stain for the Diagnosis of Bacterial Infections

First devised by Hans Christian Gram during the late nineteenth century, the Gram stain can be used to divide most bacterial species effectively into two large groups: Those that take up the basic dye, crystal violet (gram-positive), and those that allow the violet dye to wash out easily with the decolorizer alcohol or acetone (gram-negative).

Constituents of Gram Stain

1. Primary stain: Crystal violet
2. Mordant: Gram's iodine
3. Decolorizer: Acetone
4. Counterstain: Safranin

Principle of Gram Stain

The structure of the organism's cell wall determines whether the organism is gram-positive gram-negative. When stained with the primary stain and fixed with the mordant (iodine acts as the mordant, i.e. an ion element that binds and holds a chemical dye, to make it stuck on the microorganism), some bacteria are able to retain the primary dye [due to the thick (90% of cell wall) peptidoglycan layer] and resist decolorization. These are the gram-positive bacteria which are purple in color. Gram-negative bacteria have a thin peptidoglycan layer that allows primary stain to wash out by the action of decolorizer and are stained by the counterstain and are pink in color.

Preparation of Smear for Gram Staining

- Take a clean grease-free slide
- Put a drop of normal saline in the middle of the glass slide
- Sterilize a bacteriological loupe by red hot flaming, allow cooling.
- Touch one colony of organism from the culture plate provided.
- Emulsify the colony in the normal saline on the slide.
- Allow to dry.
- Heat fix the slide by passing through the Bunsen flame twice.

Heat fixation accomplishes three things: (1) It kills the organisms; (2) it causes the organisms to adhere to the slide; and (3) it alters the organisms so that they more readily accept stains (dyes). If the slide is not completely dry when you pass it through the flame, the organism will be boiled and destroyed. If you heat-fix too little, the organism may not stick and will wash off the slide in subsequent steps. If you heat-fix too much, the organisms may be incinerated, and you will see distorted cells and cellular remains.

Preparation of Smear

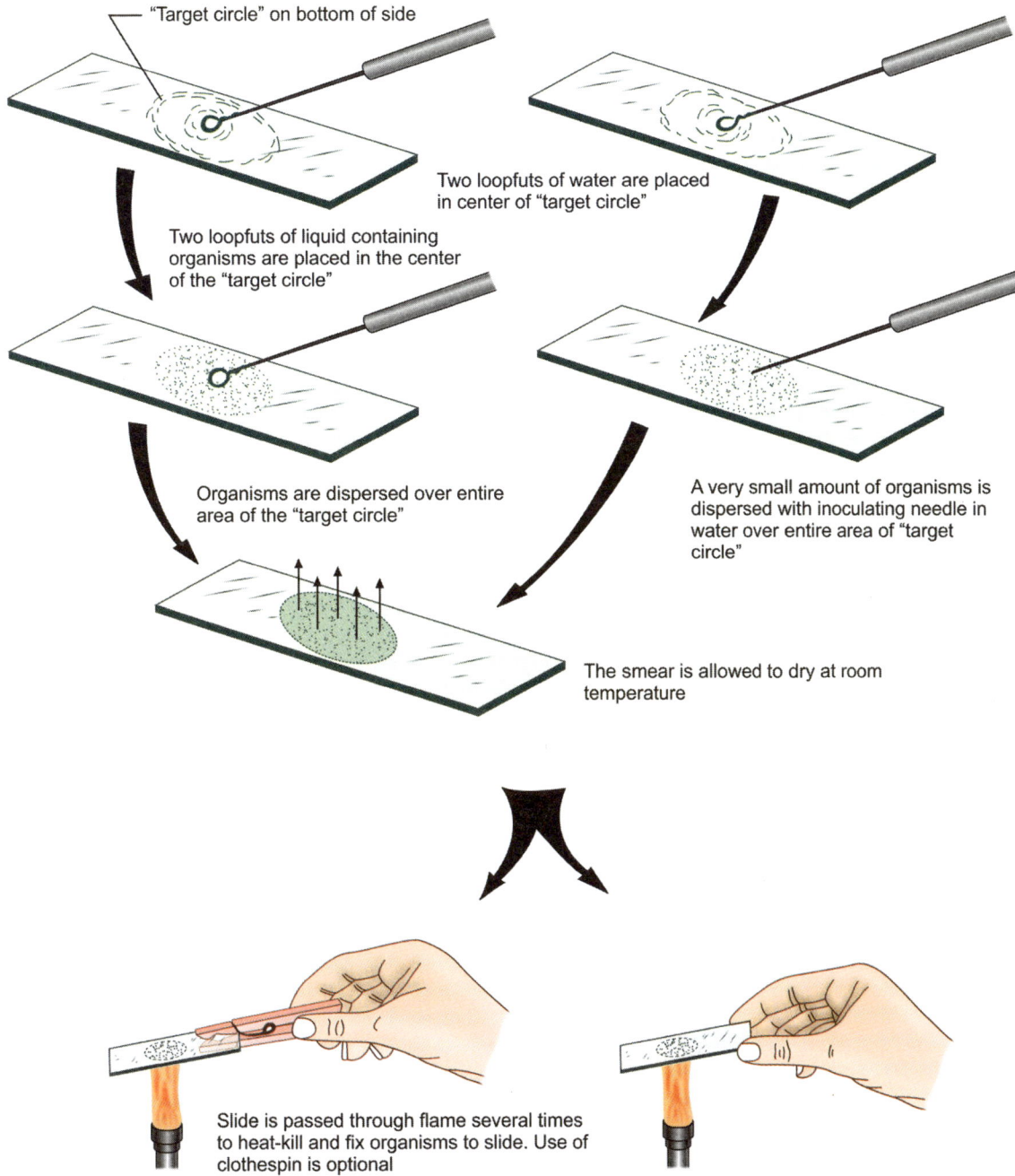

"Target circle" on bottom of side

Two loopfuts of water are placed in center of "target circle"

Two loopfuts of liquid containing organisms are placed in the center of the "target circle"

Organisms are dispersed over entire area of the "target circle"

A very small amount of organisms is dispersed with inoculating needle in water over entire area of "target circle"

The smear is allowed to dry at room temperature

Slide is passed through flame several times to heat-kill and fix organisms to slide. Use of clothespin is optional

Steps of Gram Staining

1. Pour **crystal violet (primary stain)** on the smear and keep for 1 min

2. Decant the stain and pour **grams iodine (mordant)** on the smear.

3. Decant the iodine and **decolorize with acetone** for 2–3 seconds.

4. Wash the slide.

Gram-positive cocci

Gram-negative bacilli

5. **Counterstain with safranin** for 1 min.

6. Wash the slide and dry.

7. Focus the slide under the oil imersion objective (100X) of a light microscope

8. Observe and note your finding under.

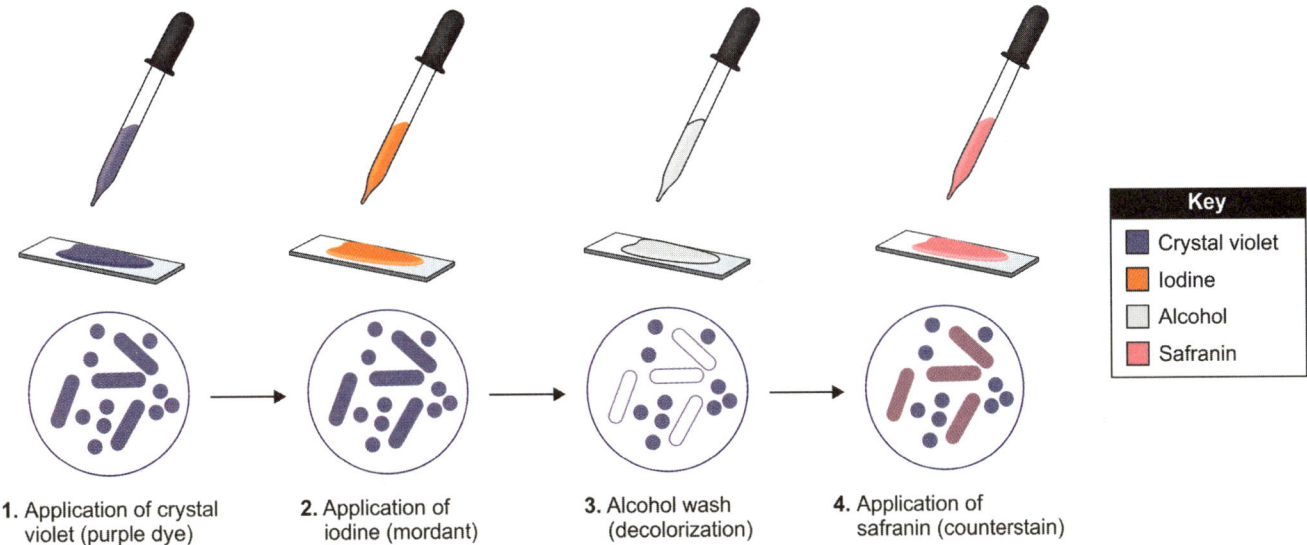

Key
- Crystal violet
- Iodine
- Alcohol
- Safranin

1. Application of crystal violet (purple dye)

2. Application of iodine (mordant)

3. Alcohol wash (decolorization)

4. Application of safranin (counterstain)

Morphological Characteristics of Bacteria on Gram Stain

Gram's reaction	: Gram-positive or gram-negative
Shape of organism	: Cocci—spherical, oval/lanceolate, kidney-shaped
	Bacilli—short/long rods, commas or spirals, coccobacilli
Staining	: Uniform/gram variable
Axis	: Straight or curved
Size	: Length and breadth (approx in microns)
Sides	: Parallel, irregular
Ends	: Rounded, bulging, concave or pointed
Arrangement (in cocci)	: Singly, in pairs, in chains, in tetrads, in clusters

Observation and Report

Gram reaction [gram-positive (violet)/gram-negative (pink)] → morphology of bacteria → any particular arrangement of bacteria seen, e.g.

- Gram-positive cocci are seen in clusters
- Gram-positive cocci are seen in chains
- Gram-negative diplococci are seen
- Long thin gram-negative bacilli are seen
- Gram-positive bacilli are seen in palisade arrangement.

Hanging Drop Technique for Bacterial Motility Examination

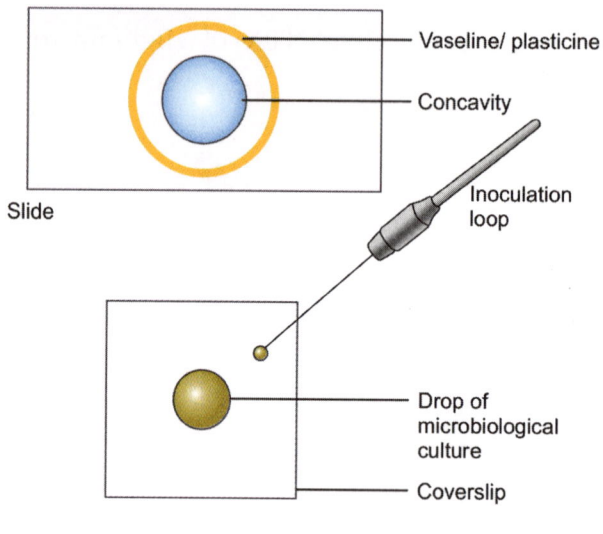

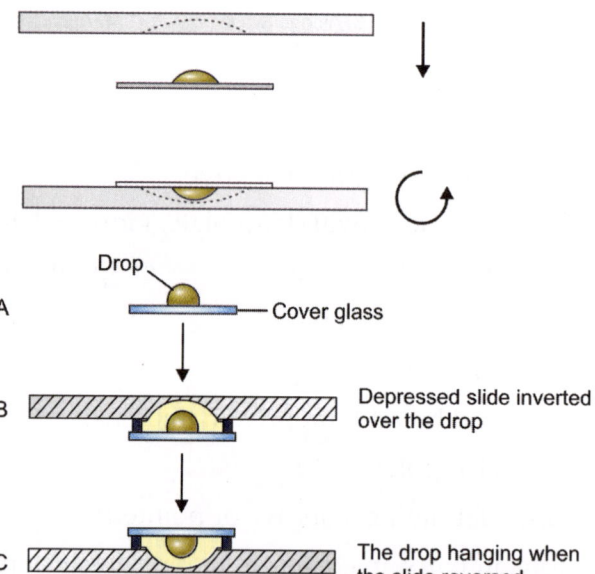

To Perform Motility Preparation of Bacteria for the Diagnosis of Bacterial Infections

Objective

To do a motility preparation from a pure broth culture of bacteria for seeing the motility of bacteria for the diagnosis of bacterial infections.

Motility Preparation

- Take a loopful of broth provided on a coverslip.
- Invert a microscopic slide with a ring of plasticine on the coverslip.
- Turn the arrangement so that the drop now hangs from the coverslip.
- Focus the edge of the drop under 10X objective of light microscope.
- Look at the movement of cocci or bacilli with respect to brownian motion at 40X objective.
- Record your finding.

Report: Motile/nonmotile cocci/bacilli are seen.

Demonstrations of other Staining Methods for Microscopy

I. SPORE STAINING AND ANAEROBIC METHODS

Aim: To study spore morphology by different staining methods.

Spore Staining by Modified ZN Stain

1. Stain the smear after fixation with carbolfuchsin for 3–5 minutes heating the prep until steam rises.
2. Wash in water
3. Decolorize with 0.5% of H_2SO_4 for few minutes
4. Wash with water
5. Counterstain with 1% aqueous methylene blue for 2 minutes
6. Wash with water and dry
7. Focus under 100X objective of oil immersion lens.

Observation: Spore—bright red, protoplasm—blue

Spore Staining by Malachite Green Stain

1. Place slide over breaker of boiling water with bacterial film uppermost.
2. When large droplets condense on underside of slide, flood slide with 5% aqueous solution of malachite green for one minute while the water continues to boil.
3. Wash in cold water
4. Add. 0.5% safranin for 30 seconds
5. Wash and dry
6. Focus under 100X objective of oil immersion lens.

Observation: Green colored spores seen inside red colored bacilli.

Demonstration

- To study characteristic features of *Clostridium tetani* from their stained smear to be able to identify them.
- To identify the following: **MacIntosh and Fields anaerobic jar, GasPak System, Robertson's cooked meat broth, thioglycollate broth** and know its uses.

Characteristic Features of Stained Slide of Clostridium tetani by Malachite Green Method

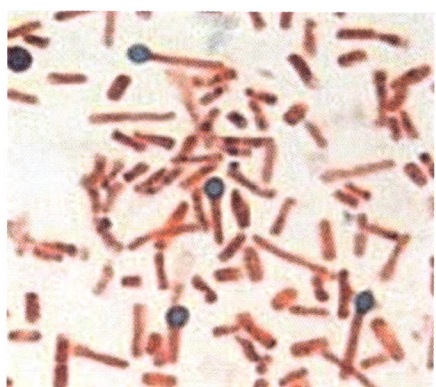

- **Gram-positive** rod-shaped
- **Obligatory anaerobic** bacterium
- **Spores: Spherical, terminal**, bulging
- Gram stain resembles **drumsticks**.
- Habitat: Found as spores in soil or in the gastrointestinal tract of animals.
- Disease caused: **Tetanus**

MacIntosh and Fields Anaerobic Jar

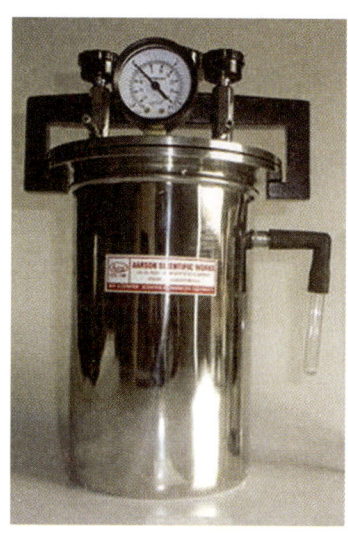

- Physical methods of anaerobiasis.
- Produce anaerobic environment during the incubation of anaerobic cultures in the laboratory.
- **Principle:** Evacuation and replacement, where the air inside the chamber is evacuated and replaced with hydrogen or a mixture of gases.
- Consists of a stout glass or metal (8″ × 5″) jar with a lid that can be tightly clamped.
- **Indicator:** Methylene blue.

GasPak System

Used in the production of anaerobic environment; commercially available, uses use-and-throw sachets.

Sachet contains a dry powder or pellets, which when mixed with water and kept in an appropriately sized airtight jar, produces anaerobic environment.

Constituents of GasPak Sachets

- *Sodium borohydride:* $NaBH_4$
- *Sodium bicarbonate:* $NaHCO_3$
- *Citric acid:* $C_3H_5O(COOH)_3$
- *Cobalt chloride:* $CoCl_2$ (catalyst)

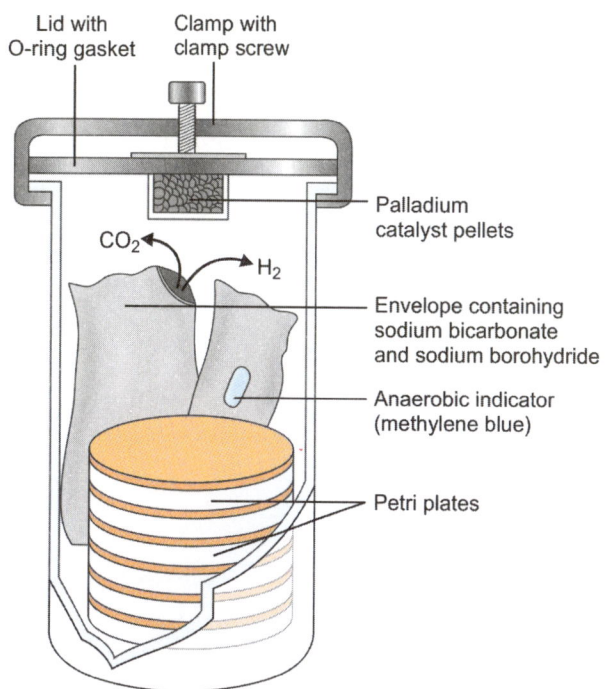

Lid with O-ring gasket
Clamp with clamp screw
CO_2
H_2
Palladium catalyst pellets
Envelope containing sodium bicarbonate and sodium borohydride
Anaerobic indicator (methylene blue)
Petri plates

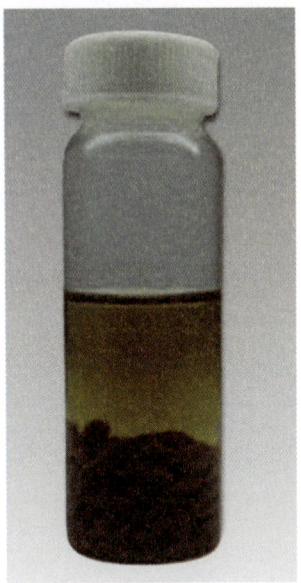

RCM

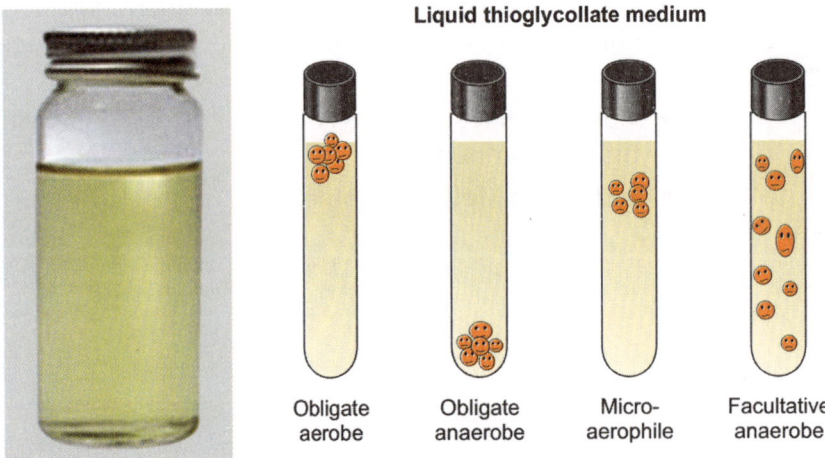

Thiglycollate broth (TGB)

Reactions in GasPak Sachets

- Citric acid + $NaHCO_3$ → $\textbf{CO}_2$ + Na-citrate
- Na-borohydride + H_2O → $\textbf{H}_2$ + Na-borate
- $2\,H_2 + O_2$ + [Catalyst] = $2\,H_2O$ + [Catalyst]

Robertson's Cooked Meat (RCM) Broth

Uses: For growing anaerobes, preservation of stock cultures of aerobic organisms, an enriched media, for biochemical reactions of anaerobic organisms.

Contains cooked pieces of bullock meat, liquid filtered from cooked meat, peptone, NaCl and water.

Preparation: A tall column (1 inch) of meat is essential to produce anaerobic conditions. Cover with 10 ml broth containing liquid filtered from cooked meat and sterilize.

Method of inoculation: The inoculum is introduced deep in medium in contact with the meat.

Principle: Contains unsaturated fatty acids which take up O_2, the reaction being catalyzed by hematin in the meat, and also sulphydril compounds which bring about a reduced potential.

Reaction: Anaerobes grow in the medium, rendering the broth turbid. Most species produce gas, the saccharolytic species turn meat pink and proteolytic species turn black and produce foul odors.

Thioglycollate Broth

Enriched differentiating media used to differentiate oxygen requirement levels of various organisms. So, can be used as transport and growth media.

Mechanism of action: O_2 levels throughout the media are reduced via reaction with Na-thioglycollate → range of oxygen levels in the media that decreases with increasing distance from the surface → allows differentiation of aerobic, anaerobic, microaerophilic, and facultatively anaerobic organisms based upon growth at various levels in the media.

II. DEMONSTRATION OF SILVER IMPREGNATION STAINING METHOD FOR DIAGNOSIS OF SPIROCHETES

Competency: MI7.1

As spirochetes are very thin Gram stained does not help visualization of these spiral organisms. They are thus stained by silver impregnation methods as deposition of silver salts increases their with and helps in their visualization by light microscope.

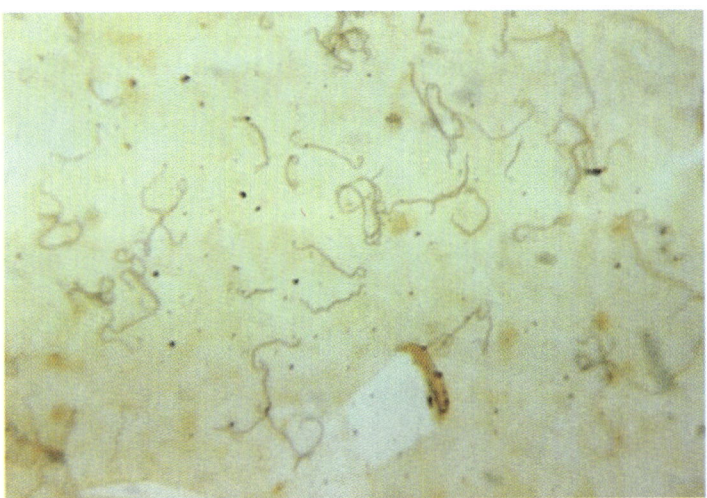

Silver stained slide of the Spirochete, Leptospira with umbrella hooked ends

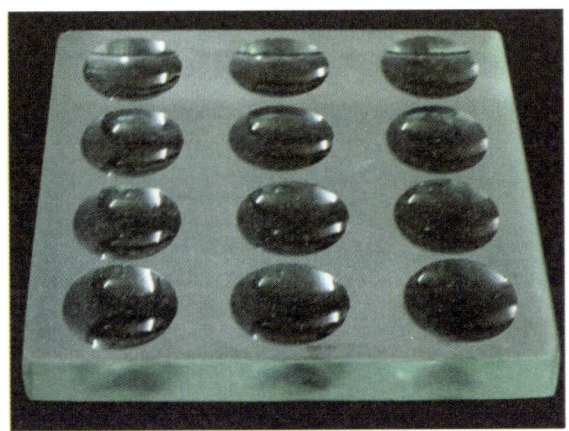
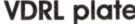

VDRL plate

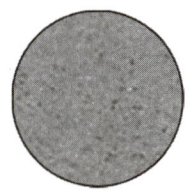 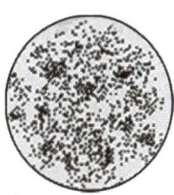 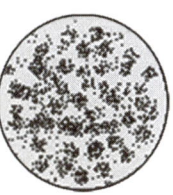

Nonreactive   Weakly reactive   Strongly reactive

VDRL reaction

VDRL is a nontreponemal test for diagnosis of syphilis. Also known as the standard test for syphilis (STS). Used for the diagnosis of antibody by the antigen–antibody test, floculation (precipitation) test using cardiolipin (nonspecific) antigen. This is a very sensitive standard test for syphilis. When large floccules are formed reaction is positive and only needle-shaped crystals are seen in case of a negative reaction.

Gram Stained Smear of *Candida* spp.

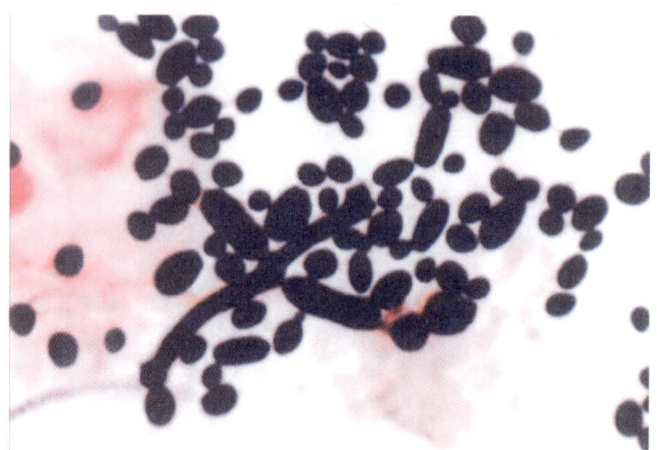

Gram-positive oval budding yeast cells

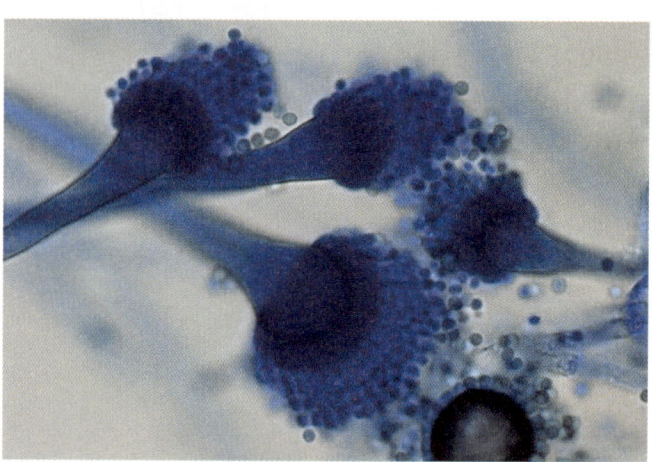

LPCP of *Aspergillus* spp.

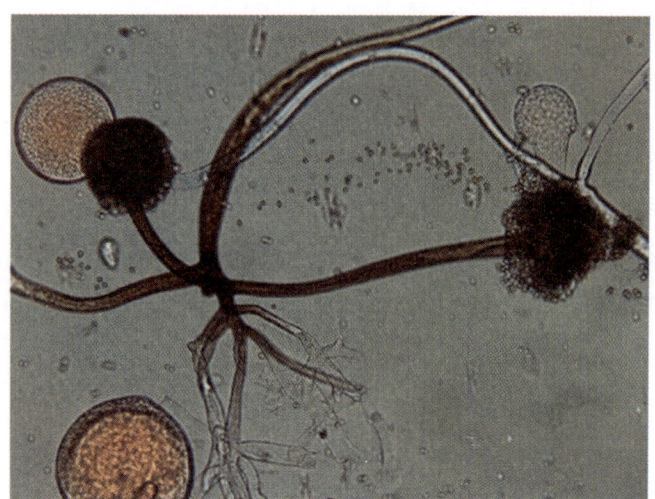

LPCP of *Rhizopus* spp.

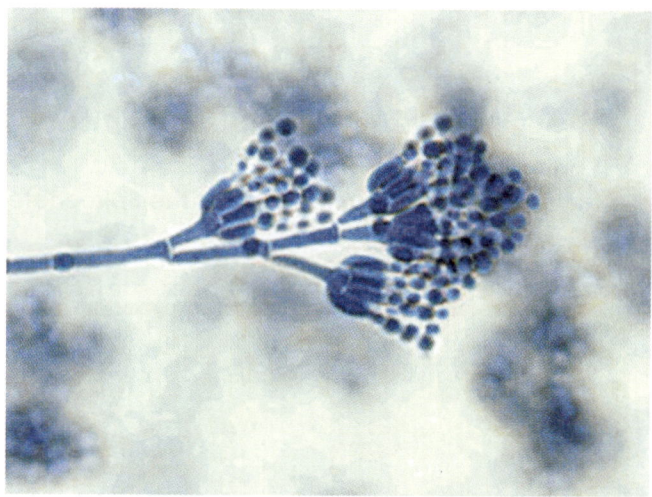

LPCP of *Penicillium* spp.

III. DEMONSTRATION OF LPCB STAIN AND CHARACTERISTIC FEATURES OF THE COMMON FUNGI AND THEIR DIAGNOSTIC METHODS

Competency: MI1.2, 8.1   **Date:**

The lactophenol cotton blue (LPCB) wet mount preparation is the most widely used method of staining and observing fungal elements. It is both a **mounting medium** and **staining agent** used in making semi-permanent microscopic preparation of fungi. Fungal elements are stained intensely blue. The preparation has three components:

1. **Phenol,** which kills any live organisms
2. **Lactic acid,** which acts as preservative for the fungal structures
3. **Cotton blue,** which stains the chitin in the fungal cell walls.

Study characteristic features of the following fungi from their stained slide

1. *Candida* from their Gram stained smear
2. *Aspergillus* spp., *Rhizopus* spp., *and Penicillium* spp. from their (LPCB mount)

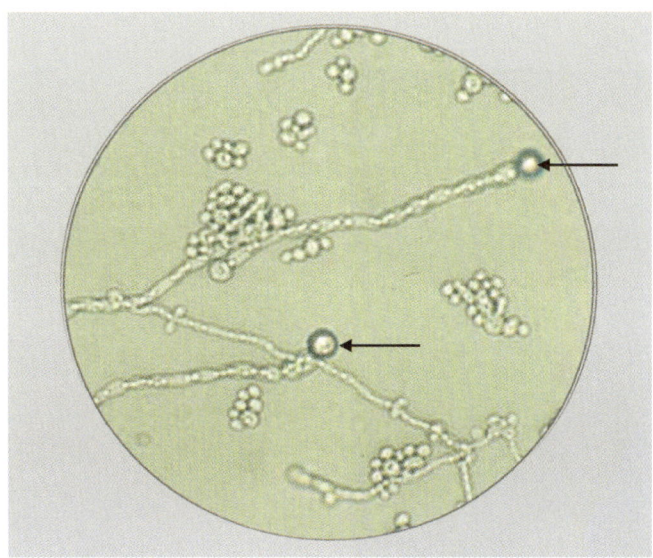

Corn meal agar showing terminal chlamydophores of *Candida albicans*

Demonstration

1. SDA
2. Biphasic fungal blood culture media
3. SDA with growth of yeast
4. SDA with growth of mycelial fungi
5. Slide culture set

Slide culture set

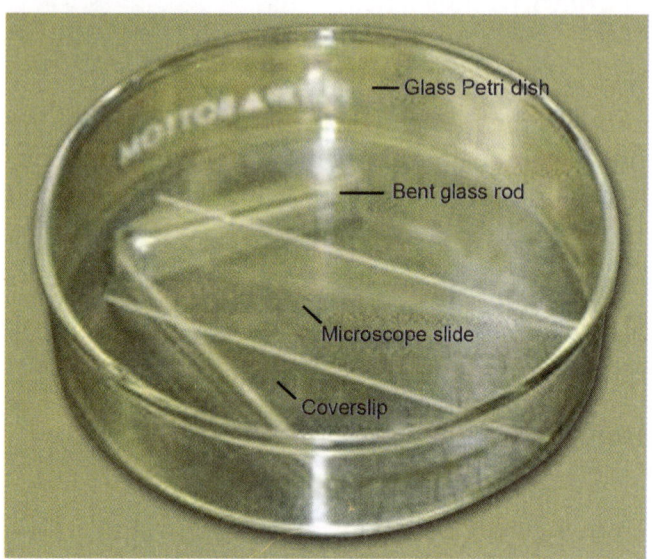

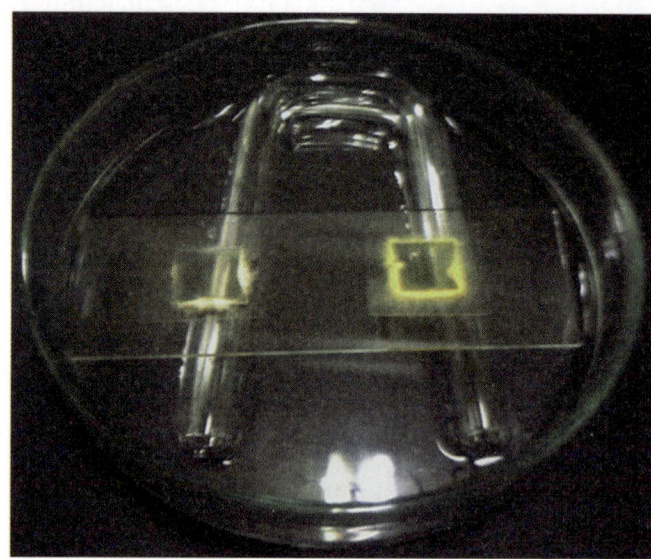

Slide culture components

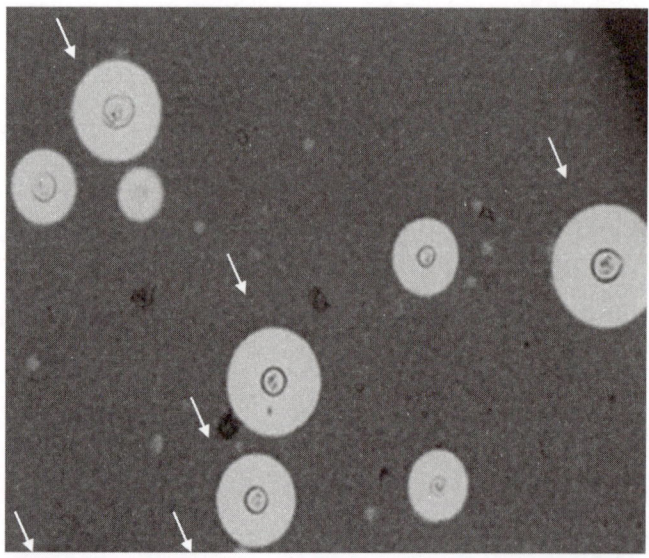

India ink preparation showing capsule of *Cryptococcus neoformans*

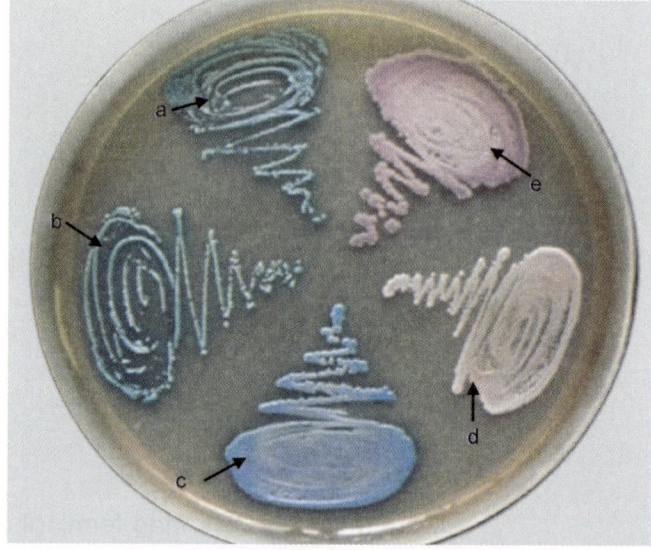

Chrome agar with growth of yeasts with different colors

Sabouraud's Dextrose Agar (SDA)

With antibiotic (cap red cotton)
Without antibiotic (cap white cotton).

Contain

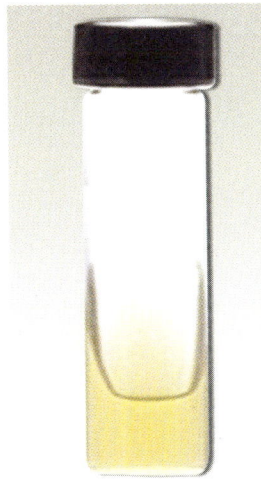

- Dextrose: 4%
- Peptone: 1%
- pH: 5–6
- **Antibiotic chloramphenicol:** 0.5 mg/ml (to prevent bacterial overgrowth)
- **Cycloheximide:** 0.005 mg/ml (to prevent growth of saprophytic fungus)

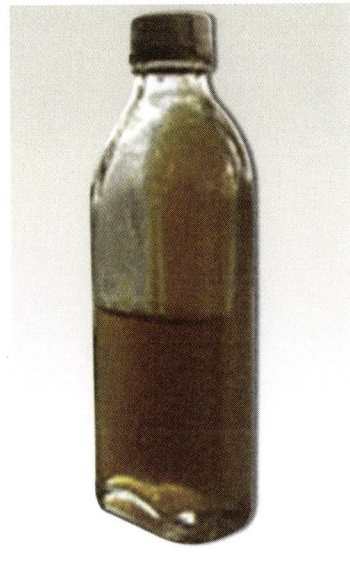

Biphasic fungal blood culture media

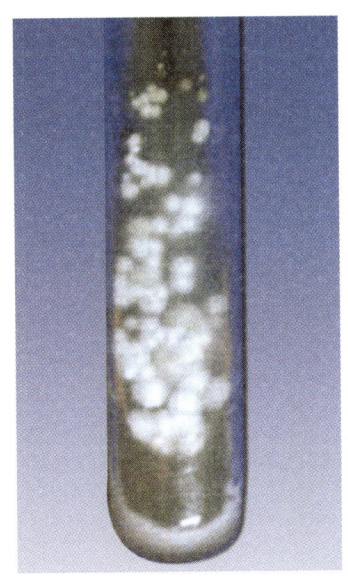

SDA media with smooth white creamy growth of yeast

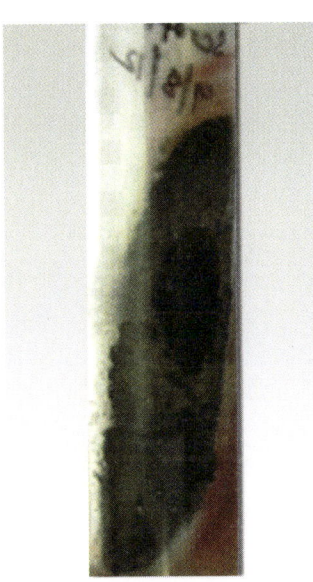

SDA with growth of cottony/woolly/velvety growth of mycelial fungi

Section
3

Identify the Causative Agent of Malaria and Filaria

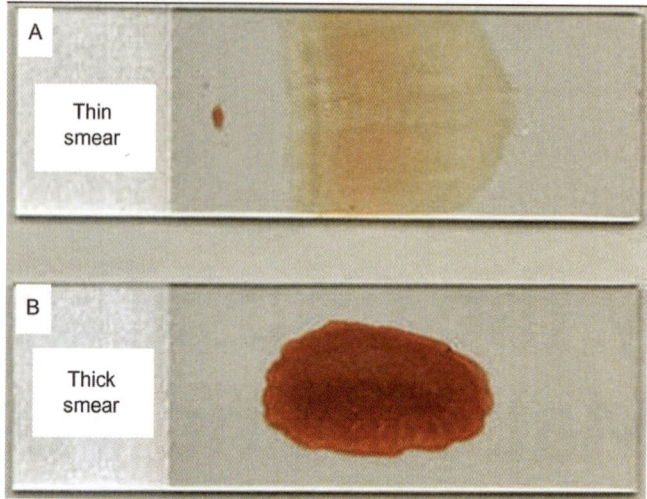

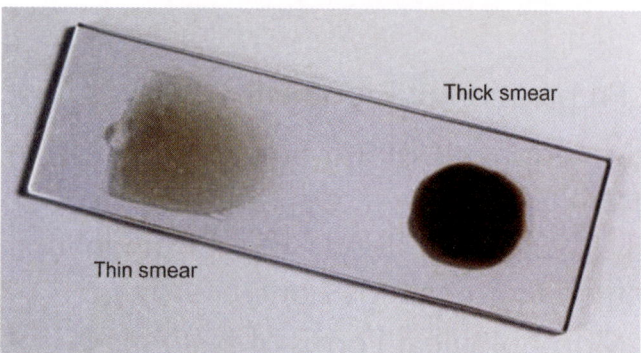

Thin and thick blood smear

Preparation of Blood Film

Aim: To prepare a thick and a thin peripheral blood smear.

THICK FILM

1. Take clean, grease and scratch free glass slides. Clean the second/third finger of the patient's left hand with methylated spirit and completely dry it.
2. Take a sterile needle and puncture the cleaned finger. Squeeze finger gently until a drop of blood exudes.
3. Hold the slide above the blood drop and touch it. Then reverse the slide and spread the blood gently with the corner of another slide to form a circle of half inch. This will form the thick film. Dry it at least for half an hour taking precautions that drying should not be done in sunlight. A moderate thick smear is one which allows one to read print through it.

THIN FILM

1. Take a small drop of blood on a clean grease-free glass slide. Hold a spreader at an angle of 45° in contact with the drop of blood. Then push the spreader keeping it at an angle of 30°.
2. Dry the thin film quickly by waving in the air. A properly spread thin film will have a **'tongue'** shape and consists of a single layer of red blood cells.
3. Fix the thin film by dipping in methyl alcohol (pure and acetone-free).

DIFFERENT ROMANOWSKY STAINS

I. LEISHMAN'S STAIN

The stain is available commercially in the form of power or tablet. A 0.15% methanolic solution is used for staining.

Staining Method

1. Pour Leishman's stain over the dried film and allow it to remain for 30 seconds.
2. Dilute the stain with twice its volume of neutral or slightly alkaline (pH 7–7.2) distilled water.
3. Allow the diluted stain to remain on the slide for 10–15 minutes.
4. Wash off the stain with running water and examine the dried slide under oil immersion objective.

II. GIEMSA STAIN

This stain is available as a powder.

Staining Method (Thin Film)

1. Fix the film with methanol or ethanol for 3–5 minutes and allow to dry.
2. Dilute the Giemsa stain by adding 1 ml of the stain to 9 ml of neutral or slightly alkaline (pH 7–7.2) distilled water.
3. Pour the diluted stain over the film and keep for 30–35 minutes.
4. Flush the slide in running tap water and examine the dried slide under oil immersion objective.

Staining Method (Thick Film)

De-hemoglobinisation to be done before staining is carried out

1. With **glacial acetic acid and tartaric acid mixture**: The film is flooded with the mixture. As soon as de-hemoglobinisation is complete (indicated by the greyish-white color of the film) the fluid is drained off by tilting. It is then washed thoroughly with neutral or slightly alkaline distilled water so that every trace of acid is removed.
2. In **distilled water** by placing the film in a vertical position in a glass cylinder for 5 to 10 minutes. When the film becomes white, it is taken out and allowed to dry in an upright position.

   Glacial acetic acid and tartaric acid mixture is prepared as follows. 2% glacial acetic acid 4 parts and 2% crystalline tartaric acid 1 part.

III. JSB STAIN

JSB: Staining solution.

JSB I: Methylated blue

Potassium dichromate

Disodium hydrogen phosphate dihydrate

1% sulphuric acid

Distilled water

JSB II: Eosin yellow (water-soluble)

Distilled water

Staining Method

1. Fix the thin smear in methanol and dry.
2. Dip the slide in JSB II for a 1–2 seconds.
3. Wash thoroughly to remove excess of eosin
4. Immerse the slide in JSB I for about 45 seconds.
5. Wash in water, dry and examine under oil immersion objective.

IV. FIELD's STAIN

Staining solution:

Solution A: Methylene blue
Azure I or azure B
Disodium hydrogen phosphate (anhydrous)
Potassium dihydrogen phosphate (anhydrous)
Distilled water

Solution B: Eosin (yellow, water-soluble)
Disodium hydrogen phosphate (anhydrous)
Potassium dihydrogen phosphate (anhydrous)
Distilled water

Staining Method

1. The thick film is placed in solution A for 1–2 seconds or till the hemoglobin is removed and no trace or green coloring left.
2. It is then removed and immediately rinsed by waving gently in clean water for a few seconds until the stain ceases to flow from the film and glass slide is free from stain.
3. It is then placed in solution B for 1 second.
4. It is removed and rinsed gently in clean water for 2–3 seconds and dried.

Peripheral Blood Smear Examination for Malarial Parasites

Aim: To study the characteristic features of the different morphological forms of malarial parasites in peripheral blood smear.

- Early trophozoite forms/ring stage of *P. falciparum*
- Early trophozoite forms/ring stage of *P. vivax*
- Gametocyte of *P. falciparum*
- Gametocyte of *P. vivax*
- Schizont of *P. vivax*

Demonstration

1. Giemsa stained smear of peripheral blood smear showing *Plasmodium falciparum* ring stage, gametocyte.
2. Giemsa stained smear of peripheral blood smear showing *Plasmodium vivax* ring stage, gametocyte, schizont.
3. Specimen of *Anopheles* mosquito.

Characteristic Features of Early Trophozoite Forms/Ring Stage of *Plasmodium falciparum*

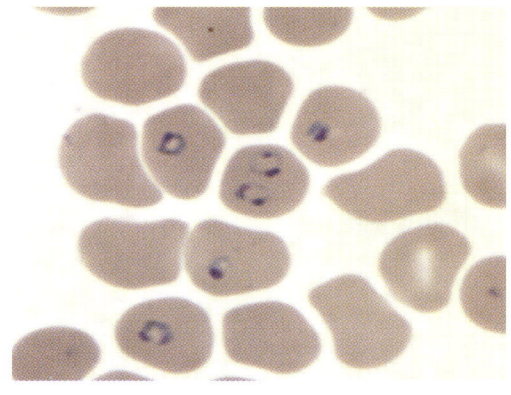

- RBC not enlarged, 1.25–1.5 µm in diameter
- Multiple rings common
- Cytoplasm fine and of regular width throughout the ring
- Parasite may lie along RBC membrane known as accole form.

Early trophozoite forms or ring stage of *Plasmodium falciparum*

Characteristic Features of Early Trophozoite Forms/Ring Stage of *Plasmodium vivax*

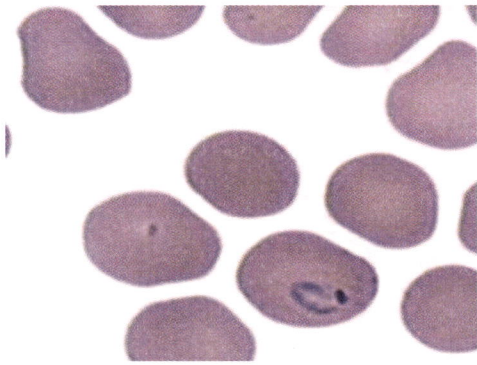

Early trophozoite forms or ring stage of
Plasmodium vivax

- RBC size enlarged, 2.5 μm in diameter
- Single ring common
- Cytoplasm opposite the chromatin is thicker.

Characteristic Features of Gametocyte of *Plasmodium falciparum*

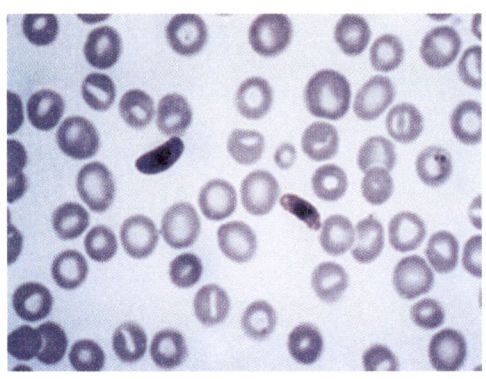

Gametocyte of *Plasmodium falciparum*

- Crescent-shaped (longer and more slender in macro-gametocyte)
- Chromatin diffuse, pigment scattered in large grains (chromatin and pigment more compact in macrogametocyte)
- Pigments aggregate like a wreath round the nucleus
- Cytoplasm stains light blue (dark blue in macrogametocyte)

Characteristic Features of Gametocyte of *Plasmodium vivax*

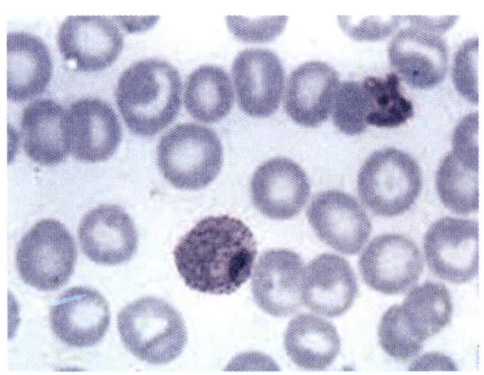

Gametocyte of *Plasmodium vivax*

- RBCs spherical, compact, enlarged 1½ to 2 times larger and often distorted
- Diffuse chromatin and coarse brown pigment almost fill the RBCs
- Cytoplasm stains light blue (dark blue in macrogametocyte)

Characteristic Features of Schizont of *Plasmodium vivax*

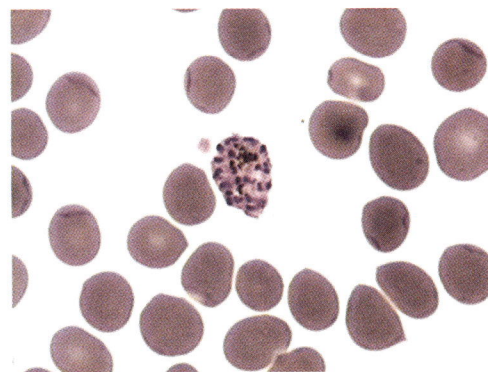

- RBC enlarged, size large 9–10 µm in diameter
- Schizont containing merozoites almost fills an enlarged cell

Schizont of *Plasmodium vivax*

Characteristic Features of *Anopheles* Mosquito

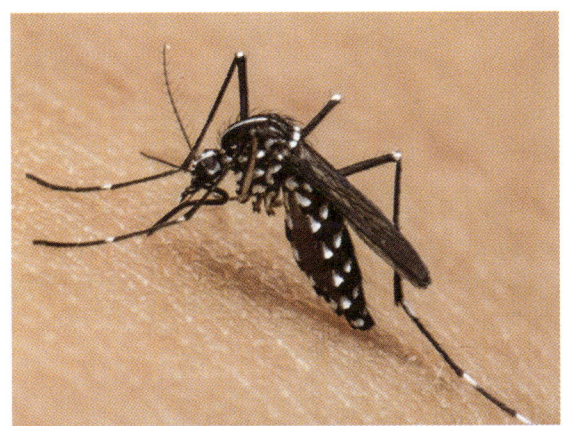

- When at rest, inclined at an angle to the surface
- Wings spotted (posterior border)
- Palpi long in both sexes
- Breed in fresh water
- Diseases transmitted—malaria, Chittoor virus.
- Important spp. *A. fluviatilis, A. stephensi*

Anopheles mosquito

Peripheral Blood Smear Examination for Microfilaria

Aim: To study Giemsa stained slide of peripheral blood smear showing microfilaria.

Microfilaria

- Has a blunted head and pointed tail
- Covered by a hyaline sheath which is much longer
- Nuclei appear as granules in the central axis
- The tail tip is free from nuclei
- Periodicity-nocturnal
- Causes lymphatic filariasis
- Transmitted by Culex mosquitoes

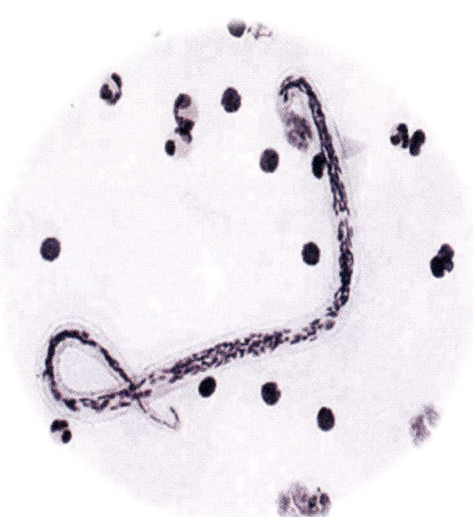
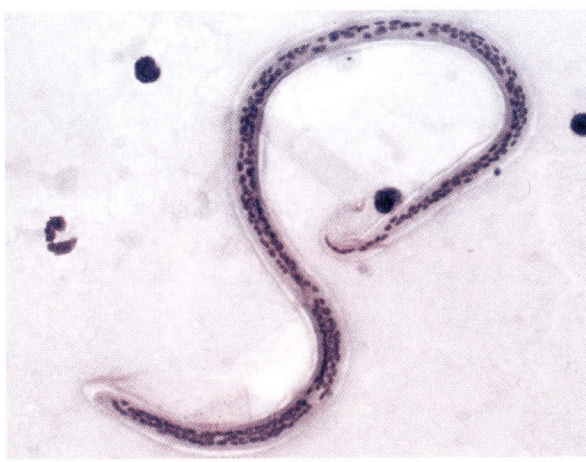

Peripheral blood smear shows microfilaria

Morphological Forms of
Leishmania donovani

Aim: To study the morphological forms of *L. donovani* in the peripheral blood smear.

1. Giemsa stained slide of peripheral blood smear showing amastigote (LD bodies) form of *Leishmania donovani*
2. Giemsa stained slide of promastigote from a culture of *Leishmania donovani*
3. Mounted specimen of the vector sandfly

Characteristic Features of Amastigote Form (LD Bodies) of *Leishmania donovani*

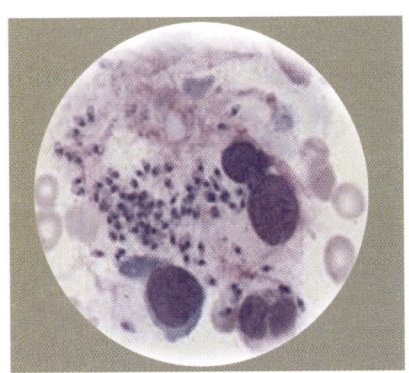

LD bodies

- Oval to round aflagellate form present in RES
- Nucleus is central
- Kinetoplast present
- Axoneme arises from blepharoplast

Characteristic Features of Promastigote Form of *Leishmania donovani*

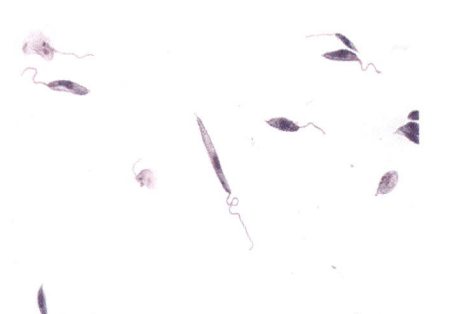

Promastigote form of *Leishmania donovani*

- Elongated, motile extracellular stage
- 15–25 μm × 1.5–3.5 μm
- Nucleus situated centrally
- Kinetoplast lies near the anterior end
- Axoneme arises from blepharoplast which projects from the anterior end of the parasite as free flagellum
- Found in culture media and in insect vector

125

Characteristic Features of Sandfly

- Small insect of 1.5–2 mm in length, body and wings hairy
- Long slender and hairy antennae; palpi and proboscis present
- Thorax bears a pair of wings and 3 pairs of legs
- Wings are upright, lanceolate and hairy, 2nd longitudinal vein branches twice, 1st branching takes place in the middle of the wing
- Sandfly hop but do not fly
- Only females bite, nocturnal biters
- Diseases transmitted—kala-azar, sandfly fever.

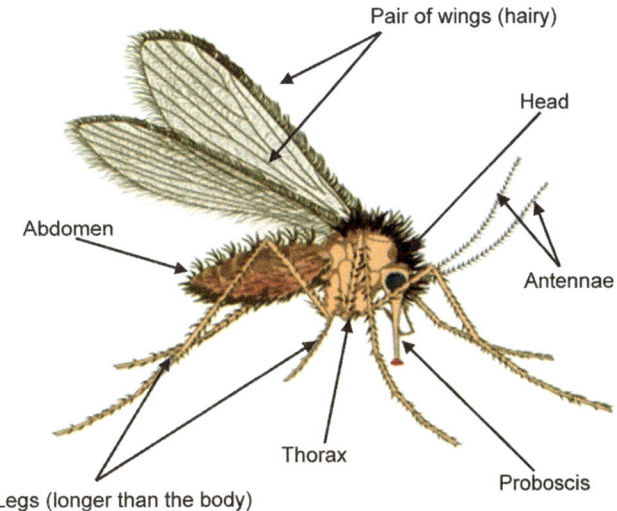

Sandfly

Section
4

Identify the Common Etiologic Agents of Diarrhea and Dysentery

Common Etiologic Agents Causing Diarrhea/Dysentery

Type of agent	Name of agent	Diarrhea/Dysentery	Method of identification
Protozoan parasite	Entamoeba histolytica	Dysentery	Stool wet mount
	Entamoeba coli	Diarrhea	Stool wet mount
	Giardia intestinalis	Diarrhea	Stool wet mount
	Cryptosporidium	Diarrhea	Mod acid-fast stain
	Cystoisospora	Diarrhea	Mod acid-fast stain
	Cyclospora	Diarrhea	Mod acid-fast stain
Helminthic parasite	Taenia solium, T. saginata	Diarrhea	Stool wet mount
	Hymenolepis nana	Diarrhea	Stool wet mount
	Fasciola hepatica, Fasciolepsis buski	Diarrhea	Stool wet mount
	Ascaris lumbricoides	Diarrhea	Stool wet mount
	Trichuris trichiura	Diarrhea	Stool wet mount
	Ancylostoma duodenale	Diarrhea	Stool wet mount
	Enterobius vermicularis	Diarrhea	Stool wet mount
	Strongyloides stercoralis	Diarrhea	Stool wet mount
Bacteria	Escherichia coli	Diarrhea/Dysentery	Stool culture
	Salmonella spp.	Diarrhea	Stool culture
	Shigella spp.	Dysentery	Stool culture
	Vibrio cholerae	Diarrhea	Stool culture
	Vibrio parahaemolyticus	Diarrhea	Stool culture
	Campylobacter jejuni	Diarrhea	Stool culture
	Clostridioides difficile	Diarrhea	Toxin detection
Viruses	Rota virus	Diarrhea	Toxin detection
	Norwalk virus	Diarrhea	
	Calici virus	Diarrhea	
	Astro virus	Diarrhea	
Fungi	Candida spp.	Diarrhea	Stool culture

E. coli, E. histolytica and *Giardia lamblia* in the given stool sample as seen under microscope

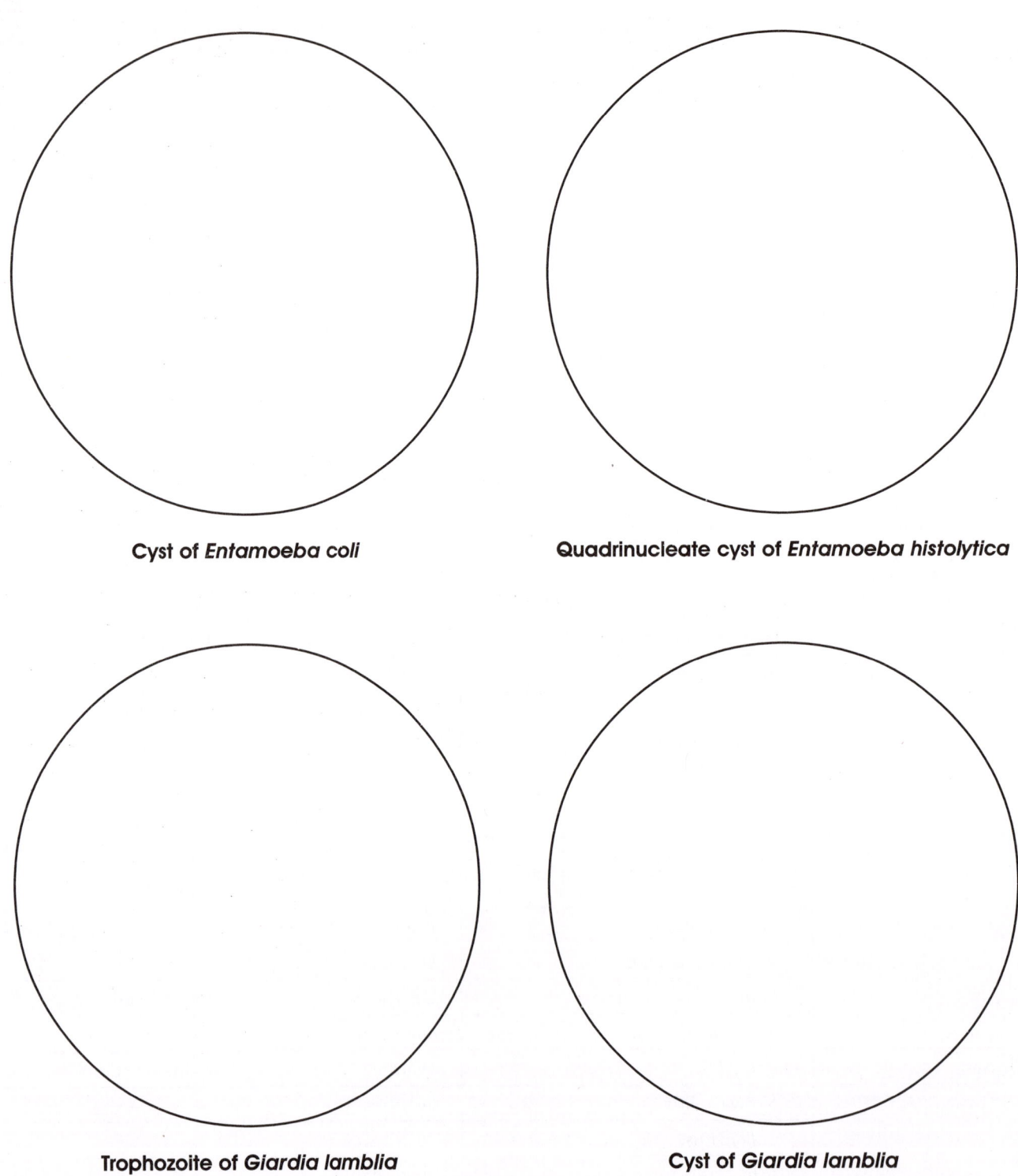

Cyst of *Entamoeba coli*

Quadrinucleate cyst of *Entamoeba histolytica*

Trophozoite of *Giardia lamblia*

Cyst of *Giardia lamblia*

Entamoeba histolytica, Entamoeba coli and *Giardia lamblia*

Aim: To study the characteristic features of the cysts of *Entamoeba histolytica*, *Entamoeba coli* and *Giardia lamblia* in saline and iodine wet mount preparation of stool.

Prepare a wet saline and iodine mount from the stool sample provided and report your finding

1. Take a clean slide and put a drop of normal saline on one side of glass slide and of iodine on other side.

2. By the help of separate sticks, mix the stool sample in both.

3. Put coverslip over both drops by making an angle of 45° with slide so that bubble formation is prevented.

4. Focus the slide of normal saline under 10X followed by 40X objective of a light microscope.

5. The slides are scanned in a zig-zag (Z) manner to cover the entire length of coverslip.

6. Observe and note your findings.

Report: Cysts of _____ are seen.

Demonstration

• Giemsa stained slide of cyst of *Acanthamoeba*.

• Formalin preserved specimen of amoebic liver abscess

• NIH media for culture of *Entamoeba histolytica*

• Giemsa stained slide of trophozoites of *Giardia lamblia*.

Characteristic Features of Cyst of *Entamoeba histolytica*

• Round 10–15 μm in diameter; surrounded by highly refractile cyst wall.

• Contains 4 nuclei (quadrinucleate) and central karyosome is present in the nucleus.

Characteristic Features of Trophozoite of *Entamoeba histolytica*

• 10–60 μm in diameter

• Cytoplasm divided into ectoplasm and endoplasm; movement is due to ectoplasmic extension of pseudopodia

• Nucleus spherical, 4–6 μm diameter, karyosome surrounded by clear halo present

Characteristic Features of Formalin Preserved Specimen of Cut Section of Liver Showing (A) Amoebic Liver Abscess

- Caused by *Entamoeba histolytica*
- Usually single and large in size
- Usually located in the postero-superior aspect of right lobe of liver
- Margins are ragged but well defined
- Contains *anchovy sauce* pus
- Amoebae are found in the wall and margins of the abscess cavity.

Characteristic Features of Cyst of *Entamoeba coli*

- Round, 15–20 µm in diameter.
- Contains 1–8 nuclei, eccentric karyosome
- Chromatic bodies if present are in the form of slender filaments/pointed threads.

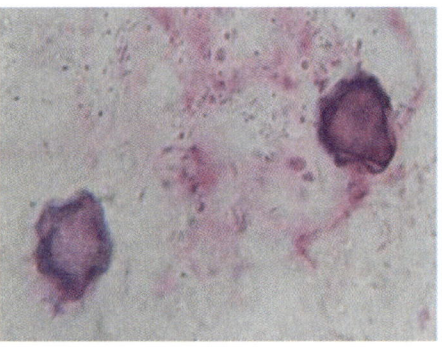

A: Cut section of liver shows ragged wall of a big abscess

Characteristic Features of Cyst of *Acanthamoeba* (B)

- Polygonal/spherical 15–20 µm in diameter
- Double layered cyst wall with central nucleus and large dense karyosome
- Outer wall/ectocyst is wrinkled
- Inner wall/endocyst smooth with pores

Characteristic Features of Cyst of *Giardia lamblia*

- Oval shaped 10–12 µm long and >7–10 µm broad
- Contain 4 nuclei.
- The axostyles diagonally form a division line within the cyst wall.

B: Giemsa stained cysts of *Acanthamoeba*

Characteristic Features of Trophozoites of *Giardia lamblia* (C)

- Pear shaped, anteriorly rounded, posteriorly tapering
- 10–12 µm in length, 5–15 µm in width
- Bilaterally symmetrical
- 1 pair of nuclei on each side
- 1 pair of parabasal bodies on axostyles
- 4 pairs of blepharoplasts and flagella.

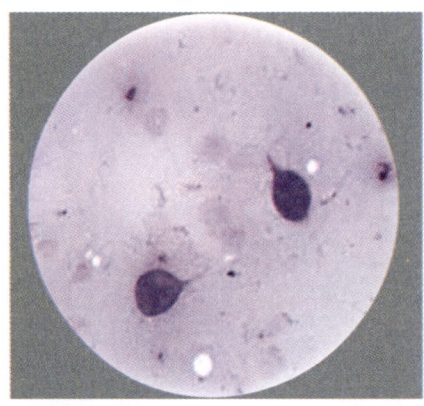

C: Giemsa stained trophozoites of *Giardia lamblia*

Eggs of *H. nana* and *Taenia* species from stool as seen under microscope

Egg of *Hymenolepis nana*

Egg of *Taenia* spp.

Eggs of Helminths (Cestodes)

Aim: To study the characteristic features of the eggs of cestodes in saline and iodine wet mount preparation of stool.

Prepare a wet saline and iodine mount from the stool sample provided and report your finding.

1. Take a clean slide and put a drop of normal saline on one side of glass slide and of iodine on other side.
2. By the help of separate sticks, mix the stool sample in both.
3. Put the coverslip over both drops by making an angle of 45° with slide so that bubble formation is prevented.
4. Focus the slide of normal saline under 10X followed by 40X of a light microscope.
5. The slides are scanned in a zig-zag (Z) manner to cover the entire length of coverslip.
6. Observe and note your findings.

Report: Eggs of _____ are seen.

Characteristic Features of Egg of *Hymenolepis nana*

- Spherical/oval, measuring 30–45 µm in diameter
- There are two distinct membranes:

    a. Outer membrane: Thin and colorless.

    b. Inner membrane: Encloses an oncosphere with 3 pairs of hooklets.

- Polar filament emanating from little knobs at either end of embryophore
- Floats on saturated solution of common salt.

Characteristic Features of Egg of *Taenia* spp.

- Spherical and brown colored as bile stained
- 31 to 43 µm diameter.
- Embryophore is brown, thick walled and radially striated.
- Contains a hexacanth embryo (oncosphere) with 3 pairs of hooklets.
- Does not float in saturated solution of common salt.

Demonstration

1. Specimen of an adult tapeworm
2. Scolex of *Taenia* mounted on slide
3. Gravid proglottid of *Taenia* mounted on slide
4. Specimen of *Fasciola hepatica*

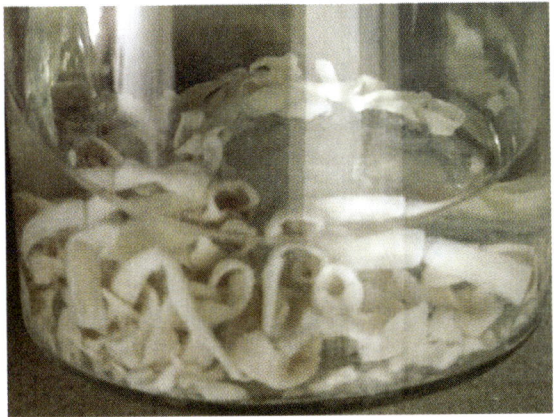

1. Specimen of tapeworm

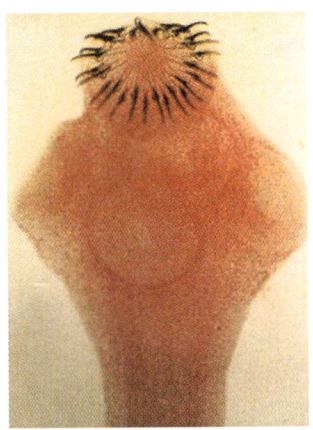

2. Characteristic features of scolex of *Taenia*: Globular in shape with 4 suckers and rounded rostellum armed with double rows of 22 to 36 large and small hooks

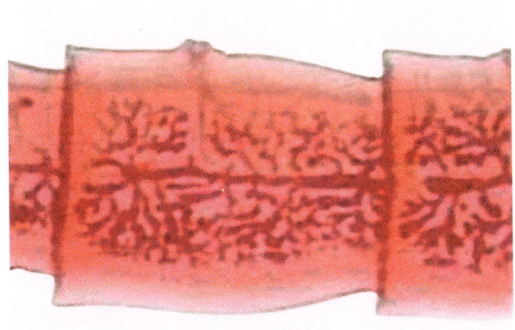

3. Gravid proglottid of *Taenia solium*

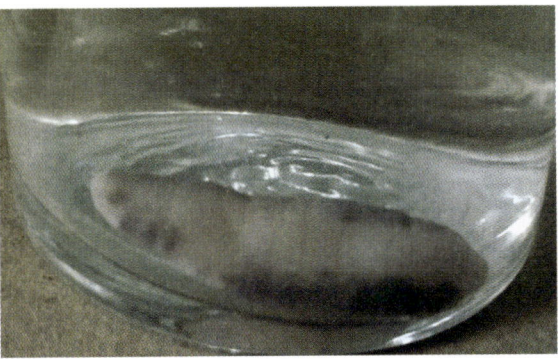

4. Specimen of *Fasciola hepatica*

Eggs of nematodes from stool as seen under microscope

Fertilized egg of *Ascaris lumbricoides*

Unfertilized egg of *Ascaris lumbricoides*

Egg of *Ancylostoma duodenale*

Egg of *Trichuris trichiura*

Eggs of Helminths (Nematodes)

Aim: To study the characteristic features of the eggs of intestinal nematodes (*Ascaris lumbricoides, Ancylostoma duodenale and Trichuris trichiura*) in saline and iodine wet mount preparation of stool.

Prepare a wet saline and iodine mount from the stool sample provided and report your finding

1. Take a clean slide and put a drop of normal saline on one side of glass slide and of iodine on other side.
2. By the help of separate sticks, mix the stool sample in both.
3. Put the coverslip over both drops by making an angle of 45° with slide so that bubble formation is prevented.
4. Focus the slide of normal saline under 10X followed by 40X of a light microscope.
5. The slides are scanned in a zig-zag (Z) manner to cover the entire length of coverslip.
6. Observe and note your findings.

Report: Eggs/ova are seen. Report whether bile stained or nonbile stained.

Characteristic Features of Egg of *Trichuris trichiura*

- Size 50 μm in length and 25 μm in breadth.
- Color is brown, has a double shell. The outer one is bile stained.
- Barrel shaped with a mucous plug at each hole.
- Contain an unsegmented ovum.

Characteristic Features of Egg of *Ascaris lumbricoides*

- Round/oval in shape 60–75 μm in length by 40–55 μm in breadth.
- Bile stained and brown in color.
- Surrounded by thick transparent shell.
- Contain large conspicuous unsegmented ovum with crescentic space at each pole (fertilized egg). In unfertilized egg ovum is atrophied.

Characteristic Features of Egg of *Ancylostoma duodenale*

- Eggs are oval/elliptical measuring 60 μm in length and 40 μm in width.
- Not bile stained surrounded by thin transparent hyaline shell.
- They possess a segmented ovum with usually four blastomeres.
- There is a clear space below ovum segment and the eggshell.
- Egg floats in saturated salt solution.

Demonstration

1. Mounted slide of egg of *Enterobius vermicularis* (thread/pinworm)
2. Mounted slide of adult *Trichuris trichiura* (whipworm)
3. Specimen of *Dracunculus medinensis* (guinea worm)
4. Specimen of *Ascaris lumbricoides* (roundworm)
5. NIH swab

Characteristic Features of Egg of *Enterobius vermicularis*

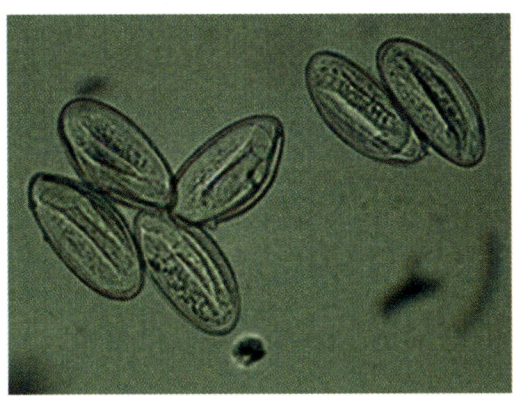

Eggs of *Enterobius vermicularis*

- Nonbile stained
- Asymmetrical in shape being plano-convex, i.e. flattened on one side and convex on outer side.
- Measures about 50–60 μm × 30 μm.
- Surrounded by transparent shell contains a coated tadpole like larva.

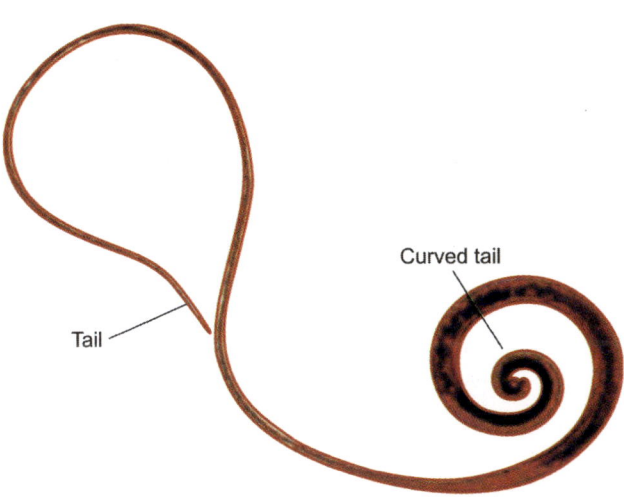

Tail

Curved tail

Adult male *Trichuris trichiura*

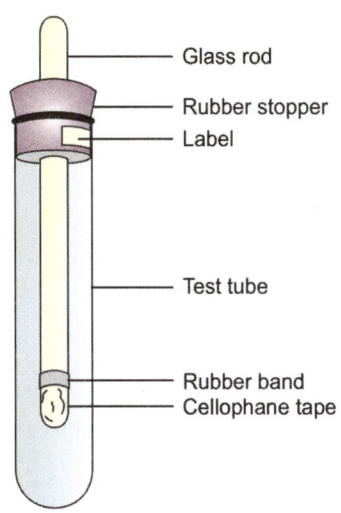

Glass rod

Rubber stopper

Label

Test tube

Rubber band

Cellophane tape

NIH swab

Characteristic Features of Microfilaria (tissue nematode in Giemsa stained slide of peripheral blood)
- It has a blunted head and pointed tail which is much longer and covered by a hyaline sheath. Nuclei appear as granules in the central axis.
- The tail tip is free from nuclei.
- Periodicity-nocturnal
- Causes lymphatic filariasis transmitted by Culex mosquitoes.

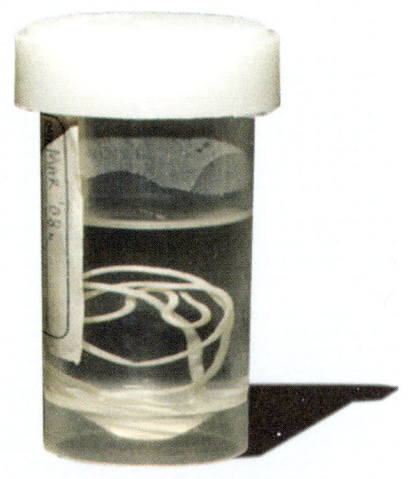

Specimen of guineaworm

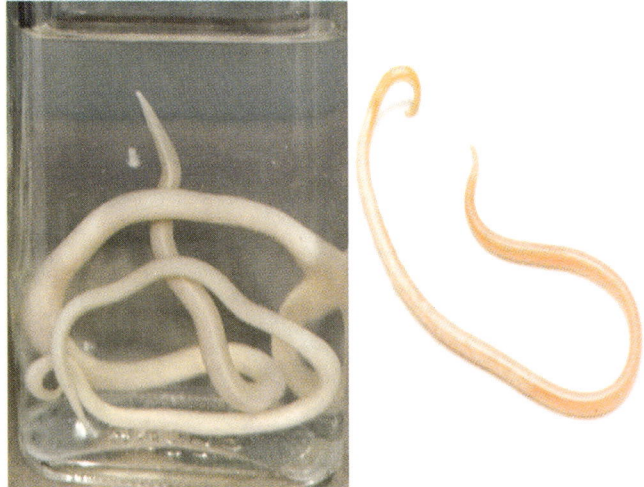

Specimen of roundworm

To Study the Characteristic Features of the Oocysts of Coccidian Parasites

Demonstration

1. Modified acid-fast stained slide of oocysts of *Cryptosporidium parvum*
2. Modified acid-fast stained slide of oocysts of *Cystoisospora belli*

   Stained by modified acid-fast stain using 0.5% H_2SO_4 as decolorizer.

Characteristic Features of Modified ZN Stained Slide of Oocysts of *Cryptosporidium parvum*.

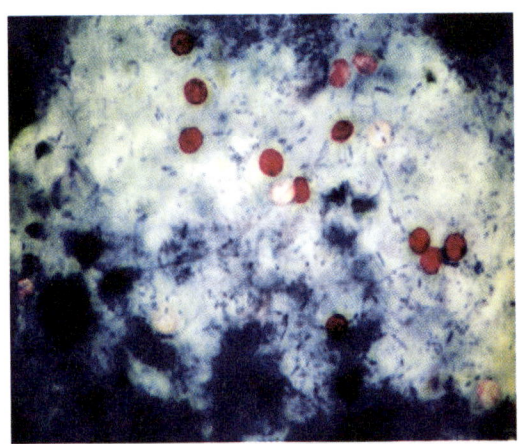

- Characteristically round acid-fast structure with variable staining
- 4.5–6 μm in diameter
- Unstained sporulated crescentic forms can be seen within oocysts wall.
- Infective stage in man
- Cause persistent diarrhea in immunocompromised individuals.

Characteristic Features of Modified ZN Stained Slide of Oocysts of *Cystoisospora belli*

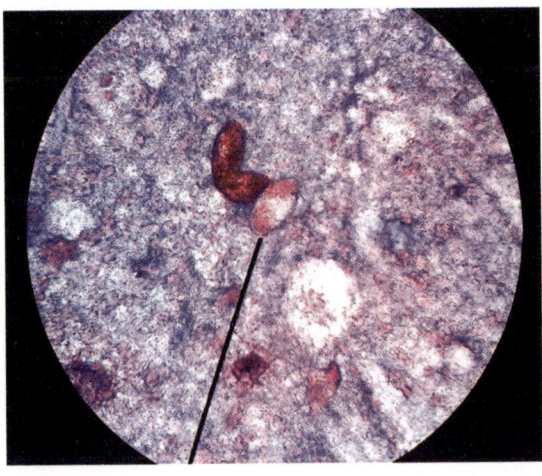

- Characteristically long and oval acid-fast structure with variable staining
- Measures 20–33 μm in × 10–19 μm
- Mature oocyst has two sporocysts that contain four sporozoites each
- Infective stage in man
- Cause persistent diarrhea in immunocompromised individuals.

Common Ova/Cysts Found in Wet Mount Stool Microscopy

Category	Name of parasite	Characteristics	Bile stained	Image
Protozoa	*Entamoeba histolytica* cyst	Round 10–15 µm in diameter; surrounded by highly refractile cyst wall. Contains 4 nuclei (quadrinucleate) and central karyosome is present in the nucleus	Nonbile stained	
	Entamoeba histolytica Trophozoite	No definitive shape; 10–60 µm in diameter; Cytoplasm divided into ectoplasm and endoplasm; Trophozoites movement seen is due to ectoplasmic extension of pseudopodia; Nucleus spherical, 4–6 µm in diameter, karyosome in surrounded by clear halo present	Nonbile stained	
	Giardia cyst	Oval shaped 12 µm long and >1 µm broad. Contain 4 nuclei. The axostyles diagonally form a division line within the cyst wall	Nonbile stained	
	Giardia trophozoite	Pear-shaped, anteriorly rounded, posteriorly tapering 10–12 µm in length, 5–15 µm in width. Bilaterally symmetrical 1 pair of nuclei on each side and 1 pair of parabasal bodies on axostyles. 4 pairs of blepharoplasts and flagella	Bile stained	

Contd.

Contd.

Category	Name of parasite	Characteristics	Bile stained	Image
	Entamoeba colicyst	Round; 15–20 μm in diameter. Contains 1–8 nuclei, eccentric karyosome; Chromatic bodies if present are in the form of slender filaments/pointed threads	Bile stained	
Cestode	*Taenia solium egg Or T. saginata egg*	Spherical, 31–43 μm in diameter. Embryophore is brown, thick walled and radially striated. Contain a hexacanth embryo (oncosphere) with 3 pairs of hooklets	Bile stained	
	Hymenolepis nana	Spherical/oval, 30–45 μm in diameter. Two distinct membranes: Outer—thin and colorless. Inner—encloses an oncosphere with 3 pairs of hooklets. Polar filament emanating from little knobs at either end of embryophore	Nonbile stained	
Trematode	*Fasciola hepatica Or Fasciolopsis buski*	Ellipsoidal in shape; 130–150 μm × 60–90 μm. Operculated at one end	Bile stained	

Contd.

Contd.

Category	Name of parasite	Characteristics	Bile stained	Image
Nematode	*Ascaris lumbricoides* fertilized egg	Round/oval in shape 60–75 μm × 40–55 μm. Surrounded by thick transparent shell. Contain large conspicuous unsegmented ovum with crescentic space at each pole. In unfertilized egg ovum is atrophied	Bile stained	
	Ascaris lumbricoides unfertilized egg	Oval in shape 60–75 μm × 40–55 μm. Surrounded by thick transparent shell. Contain atrophied ovum with no crescentic space at each pole	Bile stained	
	Trichuris trichiura egg	Size 50 μm × 25 μm. Has a double shell. The outer one is bile stained. Barrel-shaped with a mucous plug at each hole. Contain an unsegmented ovum when freshly passed and are not infective to man	Bile stained	
	Ancylostoma duodenale egg	Oval/elliptical measuring 60 μm × 40 μm. Surrounded by thin transparent hyaline shell. Possess a segmented ovum with usually four blastomeres. There is a clear space below ovum segment and the eggshell	Not bile stained	

Contd.

Contd.

Category	Name of parasite	Characteristics	Bile stained	Image
Nematode	*Enterobius vermi-cularis* egg	Asymmetrical plano-convex shape, i.e. flattened on one side and convex on outer side. 50–60 μm × 30 μm. Surrounded by transparent shell contains a coated tadpole like larva	Nonbile stained	
	Strongyloides stercoralis rhabditiform larvae	Size 108–380 μm × 14–20 μm. Have a short mouth and double bulb esophagus		

Escherichia coli

Long thin gram-negative bacilli are seen

Escherichia coli

Aim: To study the colony characteristics *of Escherichia coli* from MacConkey agar, preparation of smear and Gram staining, and study motility from the provided broth.

Colony Characteristics of *Escherichia coli* Showing Lactose Fermenting Pink Colonies on MacConkey Agar

1. Name of the media : MacConkey agar
2. Shape : Circular
3. Size : Small to large
4. Elevation : Flat
5. Surface : Smooth, glistening
6. Edge : Entire
7. Opacity : Opaque/partially translucent
8. Emulsifiability : Easy
9. Pigment : None
10. Change in medium : Pink due to lactose fermentation

Smear and Gram Staining

- Put a drop of normal saline in the middle of a clean grease-free glass slide.
- Make a smear of the colony provided, dry and heat fix the slide.
- Pour **crystal violet (primary stain)** on the smear and keep for 1 min.
- Decant the stain and pour **Gram's iodine (mordant)** on the smear.
- **Decolorize with acetone** for 2–3 seconds.
- Wash the slide and **counterstain with safranin** for 1 min.

Observation of Gram Staining of *Escherichia coli*

Gram-negative long straight bacilli with parallel sides and pointed ends are seen.

Observation of Motility of *Escherichia coli* from the Broth Provided

Motile bacilli are seen.

Confirmatory Tests for *Escherichia coli*

1. Catalase test—positive; Oxidase test—negative.
2. Glucose and lactose are fermented with production of acid and gas.
3. Nitrate is reduced to nitrite.
4. Fermentative utilization of sugars in OF media.
5. Indole production and methyl red tests are positive.
6. VP and citrate tests are negative.

Shigella spp.

Gram-negative bacilli are seen

Shigella

Aim: To study the colony characteristics of **Shigella** from MacConkey agar, preparation of smear and Gram staining, and study motility from the provided broth.

Colony Characteristics of *Shigella* spp.

Nonlactose fermenting (NLF) colonies (pale colonies) are seen on MacConkey agar.

1. Name of the media　: MacConkey agar
2. Shape　　　　　　: Circular
3. Size　　　　　　 : Small 2 mm
4. Elevation　　　　: Flat
5. Surface　　　　　: Smooth, glistening
6. Opacity　　　　　: Translucent
7. Consistency　　　: Smooth
8. Emulsifiability　 : Easy
9. Pigment　　　　 : None
10. Change in medium　: No change due to nonfermentation of lactose

Smear and Gram Staining

- Put a drop of normal saline in the middle of a clean grease free glass slide.
- Make a smear of the colony provided, dry and heat fix the slide.
- Pour **crystal violet (primary stain)** on the smear and keep for 1 min.
- Decant the stain and pour **Gram's iodine (mordant)** on the smear.
- **Decolorize with acetone** for 2–3 seconds.
- Wash the slide and **counterstain with safranin** for 1 min.

Observation from Gram Staining of *Shigella* spp.

Gram-negative bacilli are seen.

Observation of Motility of *Shigella* spp. from the Broth Provided

Nonmotile bacilli are seen.

Confirmatory Tests for *Shigella* spp.

1. Catalase test—positive
2. Oxidase test—negative
3. Glucose is fermented with production of acid without gas
4. Nitrate is reduced to nitrite
5. Fermentative utilization of sugars in OF media
6. MR test—positive; VP test—negative
7. Citrate test—positive
8. Urease test, indole production test—negative
9. Confirmation by *serotyping*.

Biochemical Reactions of *Shigella* species

Biochemical tests	*Shigella* species			
	S. dysenteriae	*S. flexneri*	*S. boydii*	*S. sonnei*
Glucose	Only acid, no gas	Only acid, no gas	Only acid, no gas	Only acid, no gas
Lactose	–	–	–	Late lactose fermenter
Sucrose	–	–	–	–
Maltose	–	–	–	–
Mannitol	–	Acid	Acid	Acid
Indole	Variable	Variable	Variable	Variable
Methyl red	+	+	+	+
VP	–	–	–	–
Urease	–	–	–	–
Ornithine decarboxylase	–	–	–	+
Lysine decarboxylase	–	–	–	–

To Study the Characteristic Features of *Vibrio cholerae*

Characteristics of *Vibrio cholerae*

- Grows as nonlactose fermenters on MacConkey agar.
- Grows as yellow sucrose fermenting colonies on thiosulphate citrate bile salt sucrose (TCBS) agar.
- Actively motile (darting motility of bacilli seen)

Gram stain of *Vibrio cholerae*: Gram-negative bacilli, often comma-shaped are seen.

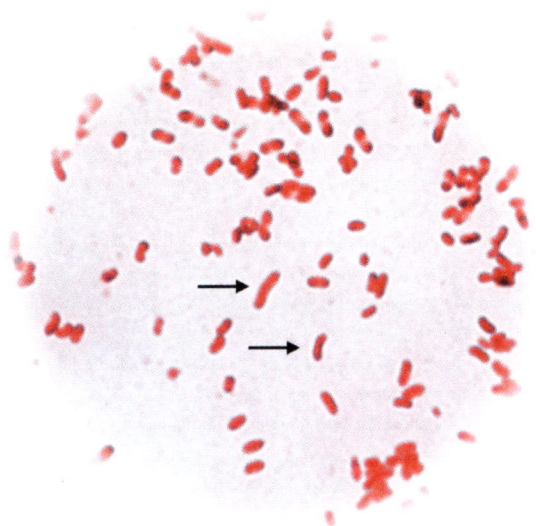

Selective Media

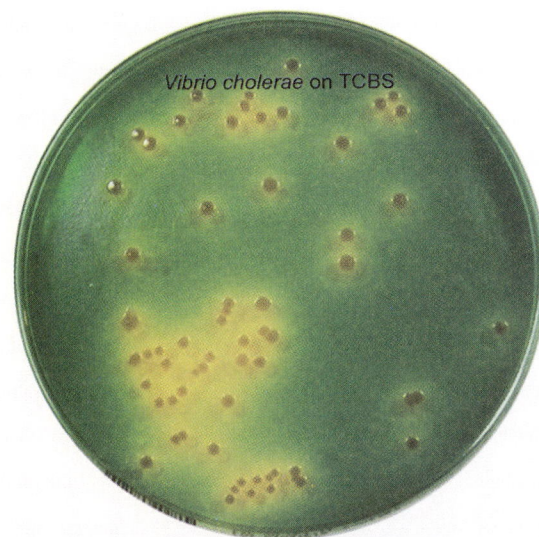

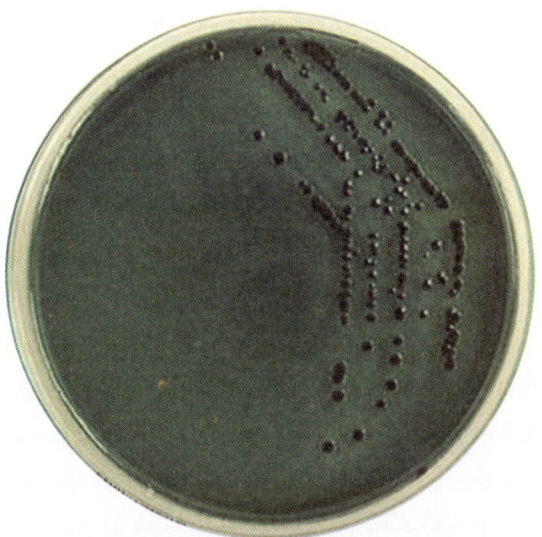

Vibrio cholerae on TCBS agar

Vibrio parahaemolyticus on TCBS agar

TCBS media shows sucrose fermenting yellow colonies of *Vibrio cholerae*. *V. parahaemolyticus* does not utilize sucrose thus colonies are green

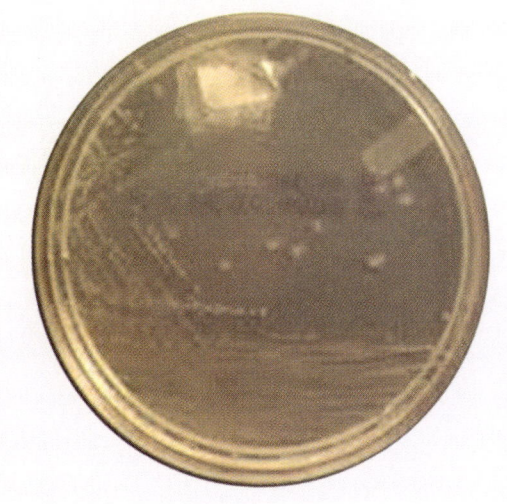

MacConkey agar shows nonlactose fermenting (NLF) colonies of *Vibrio cholerae*

1. Catalase test—positive
2. Oxidase test—positive
3. Nitrate is reduced to nitrite
4. Fermentative utilization of sugars in OF media
5. Glucose is fermented without production of gas
6. Citrate is utilized
7. Indole is formed
8. Lysine and ornithine are decarboxylated so positive.

Identify the Different Modalities for Diagnosis of Enteric Fever

Salmonella spp.

Gram-negative bacilli are seen

Salmonella typhi

Aim: To study the colony characteristics of **Salmonella typhi** from MacConkey agar, preparation of smear and Gram staining, and study motility from the provided broth.

Colony Characteristics of *Salmonella typhi*

Nonlactose fermenting (NLF) colonies (pale) are seen.

1. Name of the media   : MacConkey agar
2. Shape   : Circular
3. Size   : Large 1–3 μm × 0.5 μm
4. Elevation   : Low convex
5. Surface   : Smooth
6. Edge   : Irregular
7. Opacity   : Translucent
8. Pigment   : None
9. Change in medium   : No change due to nonfermentation of lactose
10. Odor   : None

Smear and Gram Staining

- Put a drop of normal saline in the middle of a clean grease-free glass slide.
- Make a smear of the colony provided, dry and heat fix the slide.
- Pour **crystal violet (primary stain)** on the smear and keep for 1 min.
- Decant the stain and pour **Gram's iodine (mordant)** on the smear.
- **Decolorize with acetone** for 2–3 seconds.
- Wash the slide and **counterstain with safranin** for 1 min.

Observation of Gram Staining of *Salmonella* spp.

Gram-negative bacilli are seen.

Observation of Motility of *Salmonella* from the Broth Provided

Motile bacilli are seen.

Confirmatory Tests for *Salmonella* spp.

1. Catalase test—positive
2. Oxidase test—negative

3. Glucose is fermented with production of acid and no gas
4. Lactose is not fermented
5. Nitrate is reduced to nitrite
6. Fermentative utilization test of sugars in OF media
7. H$_2$S is produced
8. MR test—positive; VP test—negative
9. Citrate test—positive
10. Urease test, indole production test—negative
11. Confirmation by *serotyping*.

Demonstration

- Growth characteristic of *Salmonella typhi* on XLD agar and Wilson and Blair bismuth sulphite media.
- Widal test.
- Craigie's tube is used for phase conversion of *Salmonella* serotypes.

Wilson and Blair Bismuth Sulphite Media

- Highly selective media for *Salmonella typhi*
- Jet black colonies with a metallic sheen are formed due to reduction of tellurite to metallic tellurium.

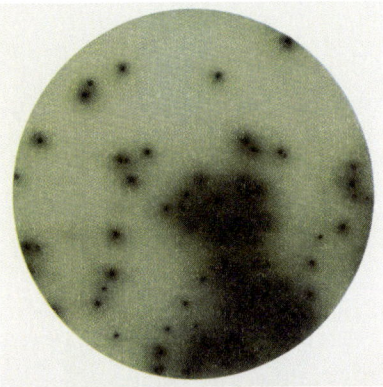

Salmonella typhi in Wilson and Blair bismuth sulphite media

Salmonella typhi on Xylose Lysine Deoxycholate Agar (XLD Agar)

Pink colonies with black center are seen suggestive of *Salmonella* spp.

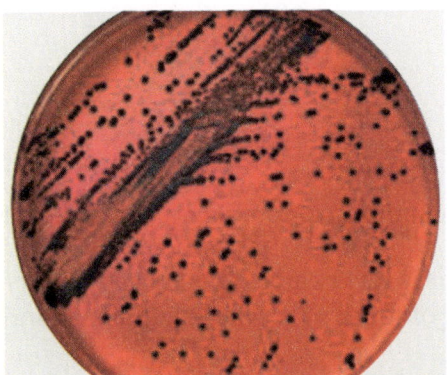

Xylose lysine deoxycholate agar (XLD agar)

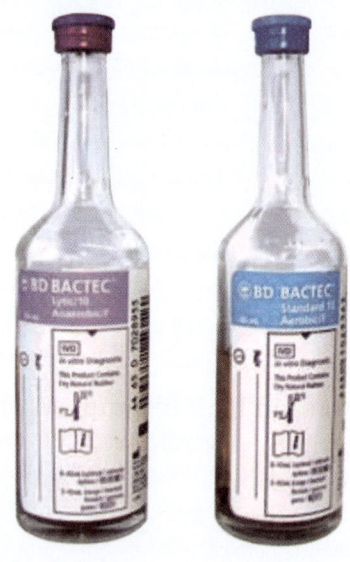

Automated blood culture bottles

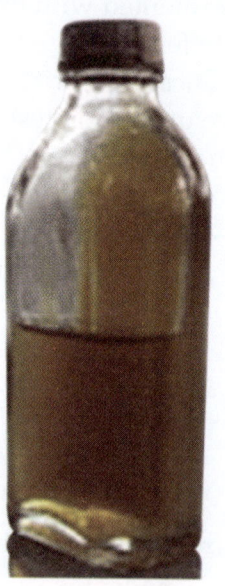

Biphasic blood culture bottle

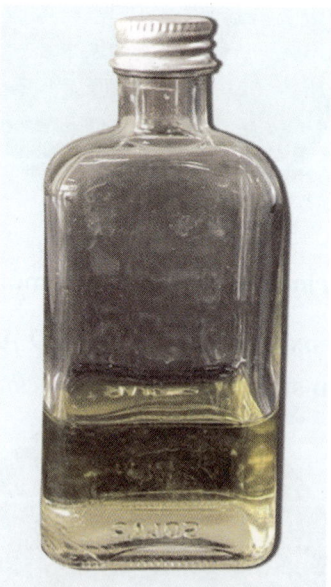

Manual blood culure bottle containing brain heart infusion broth (BHIB)

Blood culture for diagnosis of enteric fever caused by *Salmonella typhi, S. paratyphi A, S. paratyphi B and S. paratyphi C* are done in first week of fever preferably before starting of antibiotics.

Serological Test for Enteric Fever: Serum helps in antibody formation.

Widal Test

Principle: This is a **tube agglutination test** for the diagnosis of enteric fever. The titre of antibodies in the patient's serum is determined by the agglutination of particulate *Salmonella* antigen—O and H antigens.

Widal test is done in second week of fever.

Antigens Used in the Test

- "O" antigen of *Salmonella typhi*
- "H" antigen of *Salmonella typhi*
- "H" antigen of *Salmonella paratyphi* A
- "H" antigen of *Salmonella paratyphi* B
  ("O" antigen is shared among the species)

Agglutination

- "O" antigen produces compact chalky granular deposit of agglutination.
- "H" antigen produces loose, fluffy or cotton wooly deposit of agglutination.

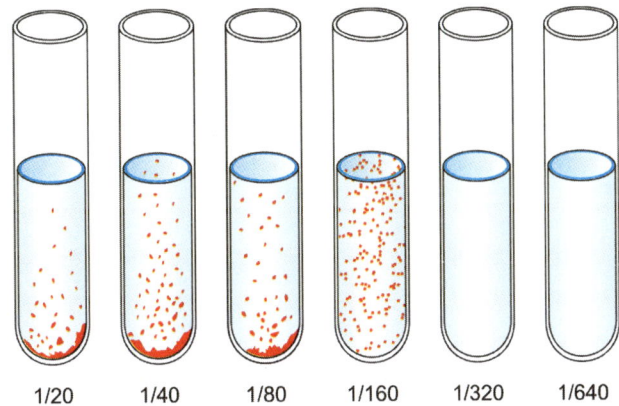

| 1/20 | 1/40 | 1/80 | 1/160 | 1/320 | 1/640 |

Craigie's tube is used for phase conversion of *Salmonella* serotypes.

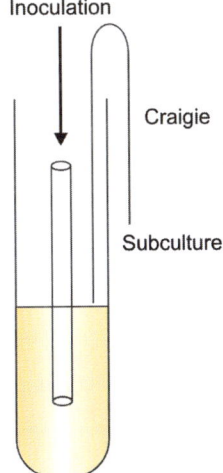

Identify the Microbial Agents Causing Rheumatic Heart Disease and Infective Endocarditis

Agents Causing Infective Endocarditis

1. Methicillin resistant *Staphylococcus aureus* (MRSA)
2. Coagulase-negative Staphylococci (CoNS)
3. *Enterococcus faecalis*
4. Viridans group *Streptococci*
5. *S. pneumoniae*
6. *Streptococcus bovis*
7. *Propionibacterium acne*
8. *Klebsiella ozaenae*
9. *Enterobacter* spp.
10. *P. aeruginosa*
11. *Candida albicans*
12. *Candida parapsilosis*
13. *Aspergillus fumigatus*

Streptococcus pyogenes as a Causative Agent of Rheumatic Fever

Aim: To study colony characteristics of *Streptococcus pyogenes* from blood agar *and* preparation of smear for gram staining, and study motility from the provided broth.

Colony Characteristics of *Streptococcus pyogenes*

1. Name of the media : Blood agar
2. Shape : Circular
3. Size : Pinpoint, 0.5–1 mm
4. Elevation : Low convex
5. Surface : Smooth, glistening
6. Edge : Entire
7. Opacity : Semi-transparent
8. Consistency : Butyrous
9. Emulsifiability : Easy
10. Pigment : None
11. Change in medium: Wide zone of beta hemolysis is present around the colonies.

Smear and Gram Staining

- Put a drop of normal saline in the middle of a clean grease-free glass slide.
- Make a smear of the colony provided, dry and heat fix the slide.
- Pour **crystal violet (primary stain)** on the smear and keep for 1 min.
- Decant the stain and pour **Gram's iodine (mordant)** on the smear.
- **Decolorize with acetone** for 2–3 seconds.
- Wash the slide and **counterstain with safranin** for 1 min.

Observation from Gram Staining of *Streptococcus pyogenes*

Gram-positive (violet colored) cocci are seen in short chains.

Observation of Motility of *Streptococcus pyogenes* from the Broth Provided

Nonmotile cocci are seen.

Streptococcus pyogenes

Gram-positive cocci are seen in chains

Confirmatory Tests for *Streptococcus pyogenes*

1. Catalase test—negative
2. Sensitive to bacitracin disc (0.04 U)
3. CAMP test negative
4. Lancefield grouping by carbohydrate extraction method.

Demonstration

- Gram stained smear of *Streptococcus pneumoniae* (pneumococci)
- Gram stained smear of *Enterococcus* spp.
- Candle jar

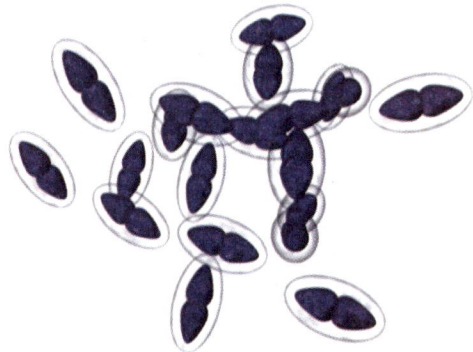

Streptococcus pneumoniae (pneumococci): Gram-positive diplococci; Lanceolate/flame-shaped with wider ends adjacent

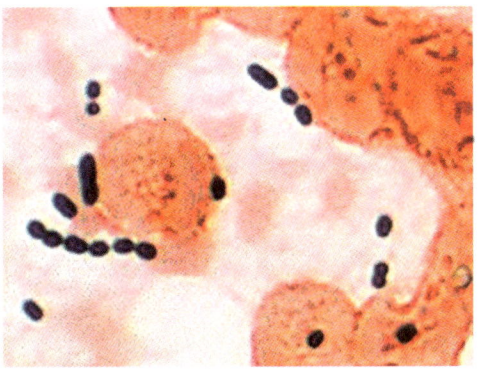

Enterococci: Gram-positive oval diplococci

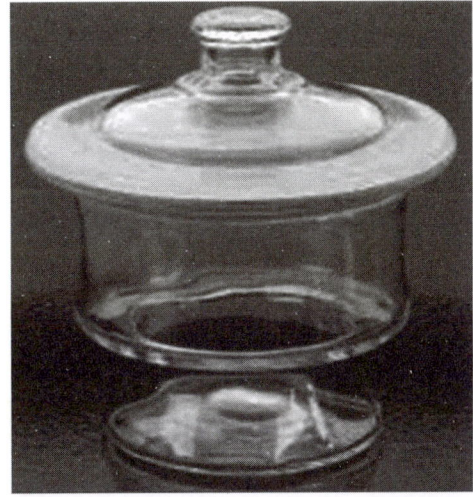

Candle jar: Used to provide capnophilic environment (5ñ10% CO_2) for the growth of certain organisms like *Streptococcus pneumoniae*. After keeping the inoculated plates, the candle inside is lighted and the lid is closed → cutting of external oxygen → extinguishes candle → relative increase (5ñ10%) of CO_2 inside the jar

Identify the Common Etiological Agents of Upper Respiratory Tract Infections (Gram Stain)

Table of Common Etiologic Agents of Respiratory Tract Infections

Common Etiologic Agents of Respiratory Tract Infections

Location	Type	Agent
UPPER RESPIRATORY TRACT INFECTIONS	Viral	*Rhinovirus*
		Influenza virus
		Parainfluenza virus
		Respiratory syncytial virus (RSV)
		Enterovirus
		Epstein-Barr virus
		Adenovirus
		Coxsackie A virus
	Bacterial	*Streptococcus pyogenes*
		Corynebacterium diphtheriae
		Staphylococcus aureus
		Haemophilus influenzae
		Haemophilus parainfluenzae
		Moraxella catarrhalis
		Arcanobacterium haemolyticum
		Francisella tularensis

Contd.

Location	Type	Agent
	Fungal	*Candida albicans*
LOWER RESPIRATORY TRACT INFECTIONS	**Viral**	*Respiratory syncytial virus (RSV)*
		Influenza
		Mumps
		Parainfluenza virus
		Adenovirus
		SARS-CoV and SARS-CoV-2
		Cytomegalovirus
	Bacterial	*Staphylococcus aureus*
		Streptococcus pneumoniae
		Mycoplasma pneumoniae
		Chlamydophila pneumoniae
		Pseudomonas aeruginosa
		Bordetella pertussis
		Mycobacterium tuberculosis
		Group B Streptococcus
		Legionella pneumophila
		Ureaplasma urealyticum
		Anaerobes
	Fungal	*Histoplasma*
		Blastomyces
		Coccidioides
		Pneumocystis jirovecii
		Aspergillus spp.
		Mucor spp.

To Study the Characteristic Features of *Corynebacterium diphtheriae*

Objective

To study the characteristic features of *Corynebacterium diphtheriae* on Albert staining from throat swab of a suspected case diphtheria.

Procedure of Albert Staining

1. Heat fix the provided slide
2. Flood slide with Albert A (through filter paper) for 5 minutes
3. Drain the slide. Do not wash.
   Flood slide with Albert B for 4 minutes.
4. Drain the slide and wash gently with tap water and then dry.
5. Observe under 100X oil immersion objective.

Observation

Green colored bacilli seen with bluish black metachromatic granules at the poles.
    The bacilli are arranged in Chinese letter or cuneiform pattern, i.e. V- or L-shaped.

Report: Microorganisms morphologically resembling *Corynebacterium diphtheriae* are seen.

Corynebacterium diphtheriae forms black colonies on tellurite agar (left), on blood agar colonies appear white (right).

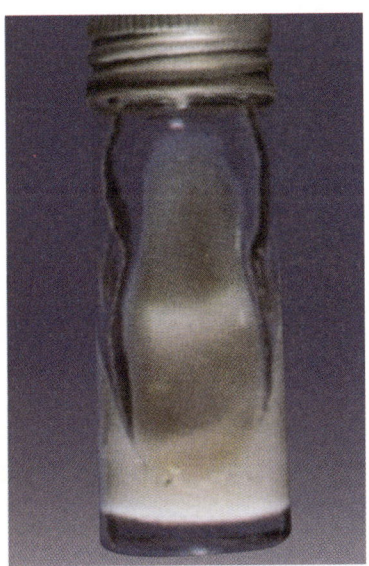

Loeffler's serum slope

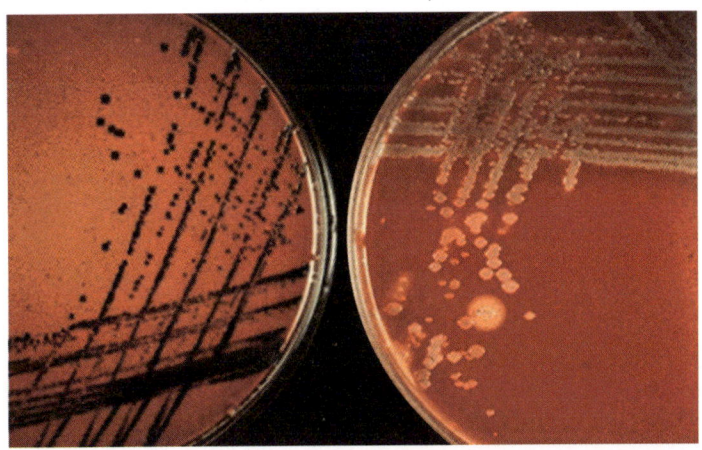

Potassium tellurite blood agar for culture of *C. diphtheriae*

Staphylococcus aureus

Gram-positive cocci are seen in clusters

Staphylococcus aureus

Aim: To study the colony characteristics of *S. aureus* in the media provided and preparation of smear and Gram staining from the culture plate and study motility from the broth provided.

Colony Characteristics of *Staphylococcus aureus*

1. Name of the media   : Blood agar
2. Shape   : Circular
3. Size   : Pin head (2–4 mm)
4. Elevation   : Raised, convex
5. Surface   : Smooth, glistening
6. Edge   : Entire
7. Opacity   : White opaque
8. Consistency   : Butyrous
9. Emulsifiability   : Easy
10. Pigment   : Golden yellow pigment present
11. Change in medium   : Beta hemolysis present

Preparation of Smear for Gram Staining

- Take a clean grease-free slide.
- Put a drop of normal saline in the middle of the glass slide.
- Sterilize a bacteriological loop by red hot flaming, allow to cool.
- Touch one colony of *Staphylococcus aureus* from the plate of blood agar provided.
- Emulsify the colony in the normal saline on the slide.
- Allow to air dry.
- Heat fix the slide by passing the glass slide with the smear 3–4 times across the flame.

Steps of Gram Staining

1. Pour **crystal violet (primary stain)** on the smear and keep for 1 min.
2. Decant the stain and pour **Gram's iodine (mordant)** on the smear.
3. Decant the iodine and **decolorize with acetone** for 2–3 seconds.
4. Wash the slide.
5. **Counterstain with safranin** for 1 min.

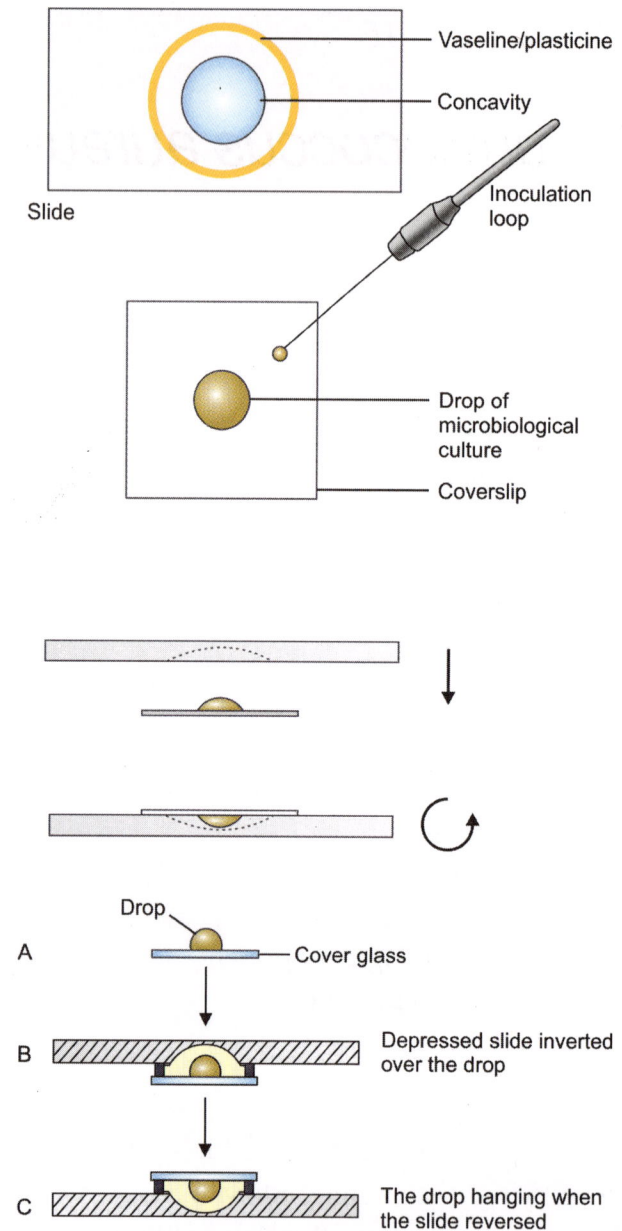

Hanging drop technique for bacterial motility examination

6. Wash the slide with water and air dry.

7. Focus the slide under the oil immersion objective (100X) of a light microscope.

8. Observe and note your finding.

Observation

Gram-positive (violet colored) cocci are seen in grape-like clusters.

Motility Preparation

- Take a loopful of the broth provided and place the drop on a coverslip.
- Invert a glass slide with a ring of plasticine on the coverslip.
- Turn the slide with coverslip facing upwards down so that the drop now hangs from the coverslip.
- Focus the edge of the drop under 10X objective of light microscope.
- Look at the movement of cocci or bacilli with respect to Brownian motion at 40X objective.
- Record your findings.

Observation of Motility of *Staphylococcus aureus* from the Broth Provided

Nonmotile cocci are seen.

Confirmatory Tests for *Staphylococcus aureus*

1. Catalase test—positive
2. Coagulase test—positive

COAGULASE TEST

Slide Coagulase Test

- A milky emulsion in normal saline is prepared from isolated colony of *Staphylococcus aureus* on a clean glass slide.
- One loopful of sterile rabbit plasma is added to this emulsion and mixed thoroughly.
- The slide is then rocked to and fro.
- Visible clumps are formed if the test organism is *Staphylococcus aureus*.
- This is a test for identifying the "clumping factor" or bound coagulase.

Tube Coagulase Test

- 1:6 dilution of rabbit plasma in normal saline is prepared.
- 1 ml of this solution is taken in each of four test tubes.
- To each of the first three tubes one colony of the test strain, a known coagulase positive *S. aureus* and a known coagulase negative *strain of Staphylococcus* spp. are added respectively.
- The fourth is left as it is as a control.

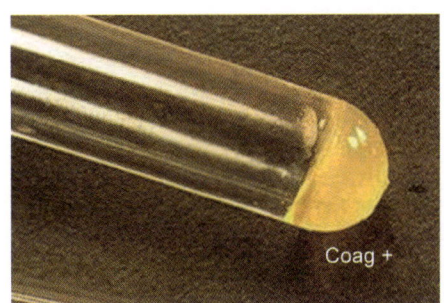

Staphylococcus aureus

Coag +

Tube coagulase test

Difference between *Staphylococcus* and *Micrococcus*		
Criteria	*Staphylococcus*	*Micrococcus*
Anaerobic growth	+	−
Carbohydrate utilization	Fermentative	Oxidative
Catalase	+	+
Oxidase (modified)	−	+
Bacitracin (0.04 U) disc	Resistant	Sensitive
Lysostaphin	Sensitive	Resistant
Difference between *Staphylococcus aureus* and *Staphylococcus epidermidis*		
Criteria	*Staphylococcus aureus*	*Staphylococcus epidermidis*
Pigment	+	−
Coagulase	+	−
Phosphatase	+	+
Mannitol fermentation	+	−
Trehalose fermentation	+	−
Difference between *Staphylococcus aureus* and *Staphylococcus saprophyticus*		
Criteria	*Staphylococcus aureus*	*Staphylococcus saprophyticus*
Pigment	+	Variable
Coagulase	+	−
Phosphatase	+	−
Mannitol fermentation	+	+
Novobiocin resistance	−	+

- The tubes are then incubated at 37°C and checked for clot formation every 30 minutes for up to 4 hours.
- Visible clot formation signifies production of coagulase enzyme and identifies the test strain as *S. aureus*.

Demonstration

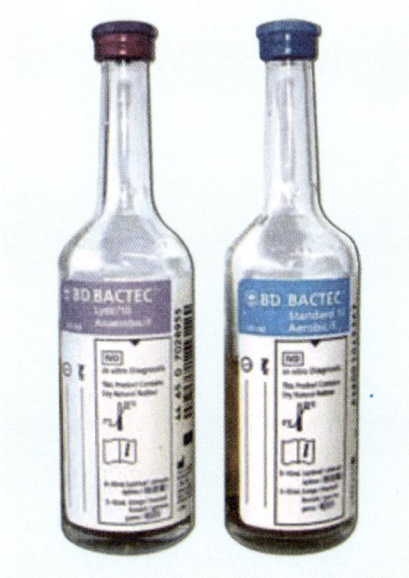

Automated blood culture bottles

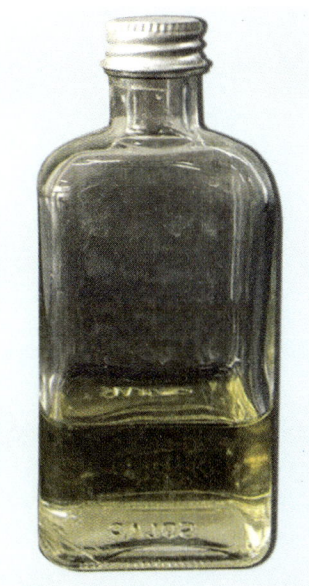

Brain heart infusion broth

Staphylococcus aureus

Gram-positive cocci are seen in clusters

Other Agents Causing Upper Respiratory Tract Infections, e.g. *Streptococcus pyogenes*, *Staphylococcus aureus* (Revision Practical)

Streptococcus pyogenes

Gram-positive cocci are seen in chains

Identify the Common Etiological Agents of Lower Respiratory Tract Infections (Gram Stain and Acid-fast Stain)

43. To Study the Characteristic Features of *Klebsiella* spp.

44. To Study the Characteristic Features of *Mycobacterium tuberculosis*

45. To Study the Characteristic Features of *Pseudomonas* spp.

46. Other Agents Causing Lower Respiratory Tract Infections, e.g. Staphylococcus aureus, Pneumococcus, Aspergillus spp. (Revision Practical)

Klebsiella spp.

Short plump gram-negative bacilli are seen

To Study the Characteristic Features of *Klebsiella* spp.

Aim: To study colony characteristics of **Klebsiella** from MacConkey agar, preparation of smear and Gram staining, and study motility from the provided broth.

Colony Characteristics of *Klebsiella* spp.

1. Name of the media　　: MacConkey agar
2. Shape　　　　　　　　: Circular
3. Size　　　　　　　　　: Large
4. Elevation　　　　　　: Dome-shaped
5. Surface　　　　　　　: Smooth, glistening
6. Edge　　　　　　　　: Entire
7. Consistency　　　　　: Mucoid
8. Emulsifiability　　　: Easy
9. Pigment　　　　　　　: None
10. Change in medium　: Pink due to fermentation of lactose

Smear and Gram Staining

- Put a drop of normal saline in the middle of a clean grease-free glass slide.
- Make a smear of the colony provided, dry and heat fix the slide.
- Pour **crystal violet (primary stain)** on the smear and keep for 1 min.
- Decant the stain and pour **Gram's iodine (mordant)** on the smear.
- **Decolorize with acetone** for 2–3 seconds.
- Wash the slide and **counterstain with safranin** for 1 min.

Observation of Gram Staining of *Klebsiella* spp.

Short plump straight gram-negative bacilli are seen.

Observation of Motility of *Klebsiella* spp. from the Broth Provided

Nonmotile bacilli are seen.

Confirmatory Tests for *Klebsiella* spp.

1. Catalase test—positive; Oxidase test—negative.
2. Glucose and lactose are fermented with production of acid and gas.
3. Nitrate is reduced to nitrite.
4. Fermentative utilization of sugars in OF media.
5. Indole production and methyl red tests are negative.
6. VP and citrate tests are positive.

Common species: *K. pneumoniae, K. oxytoca.*

To Study the Characteristic Features of *Mycobacterium tuberculosis*

Objective: To study the characteristic features of *Mycobacterium tuberculosis*

Sputum smear prepared after decontamination of sputum sample by Petroff's method using *N*-acetyl-L-cysteine and sodium hydroxide and stained by Ziehl-Neelsen (ZN) technique using 20% H_2SO_4 as decolorizer.

On ZN staining, red colored bacilli with beaded appearance seen against a blue background

Report: Acid-fast bacilli are seen.

Demonstration

- To study characteristic features of *Mycobacterium leprae* from their ZN stained slides.
- To study growth characteristics of *Mycobacterium tuberculosis* and atypical mycobacteria (non-tuberculous mycobacteria) on Lowenstein-Jensen (LJ) media.

Characteristic features of *Mycobacterium leprae* from their AFB stained slides of a slit skin smear using 5% H_2SO_4 as decolorizer:

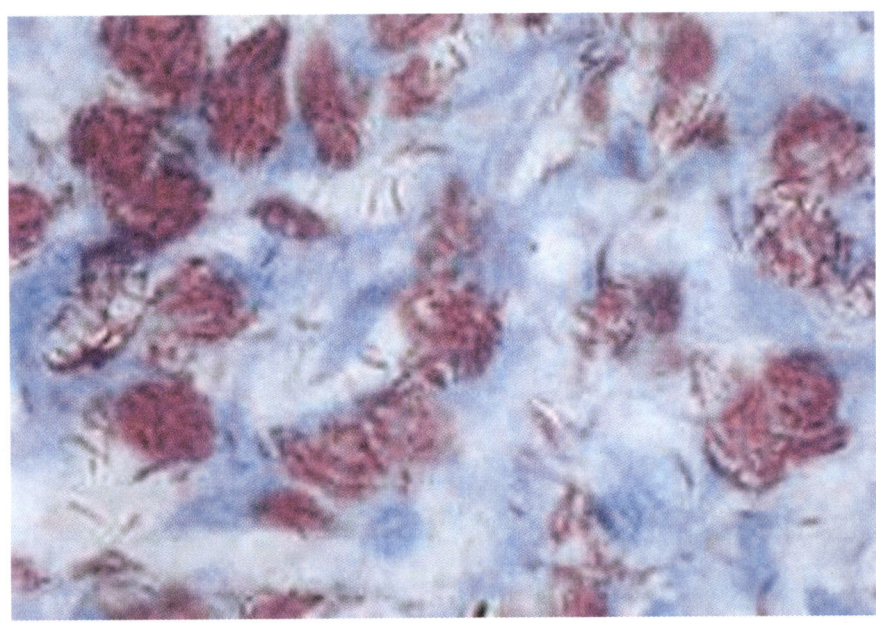

Red colored bacilli with beaded appearance are seen in globi or clumps

Mycobacterium leprae is uncultivable in artificial culture media but can only be maintained in the following animals

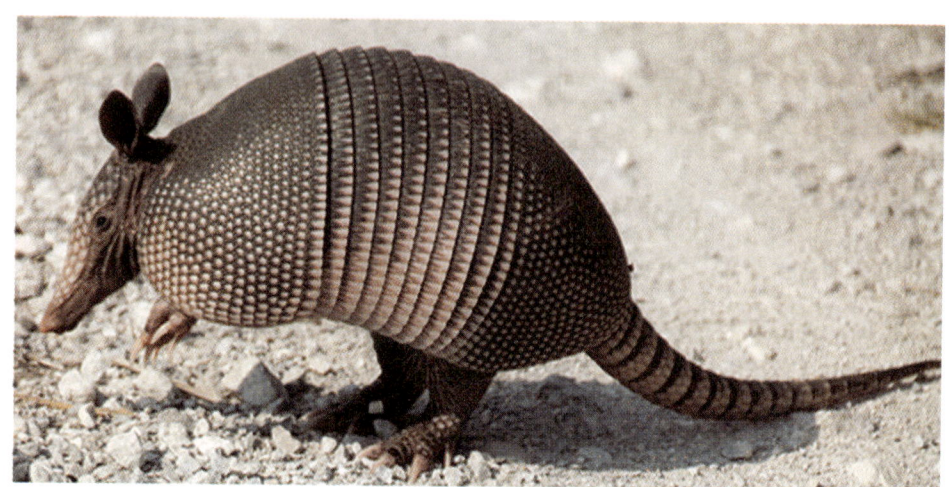

9-banded armadillo

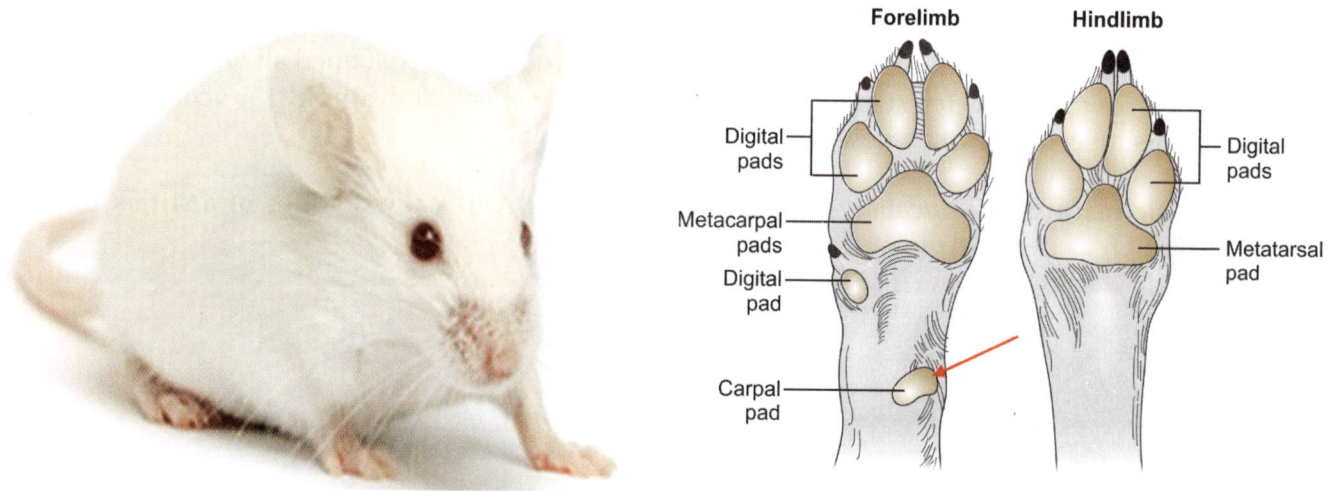

Mouse foot pad

Growth characteristics of *Mycobacterium tuberculosis* and atypical mycobacteria (NTM) on LJ medium:

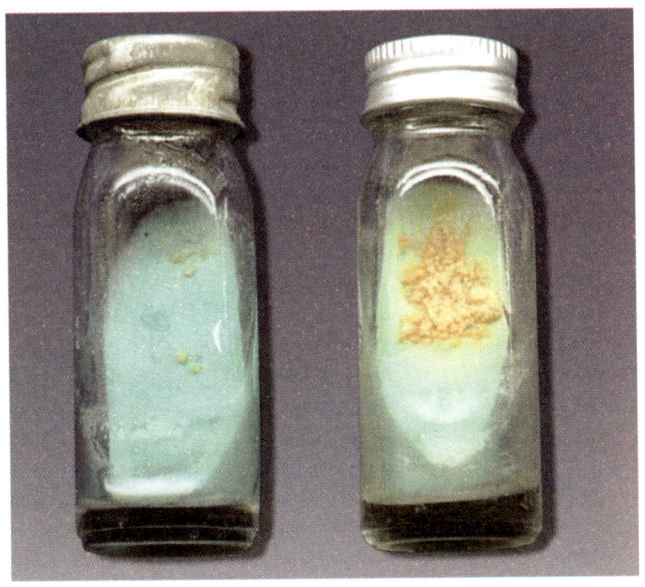

- *Mycobacterium tuberculosis* growth appears as **rough, tough and buff** colored colonies against the green background of the LJ media.
- Atypical mycobacteria on LJ medium grows as yellow pigmented colonies against the green background of the LJ media.

Constituents of LJ Medium

L-Asparagine (sources of nitrogen and vitamins)

Monopotassium phosphate and **magnesium sulfate** enhance organism growth and act as buffers.

Malachite green (act as selective agent)

Egg (provide fatty acids and protein for the metabolism of mycobacteria and solidifying agent)

Glycerol is carbon source and favorable to the growth of the human type tubercle bacillus while being unfavorable to the bovine type. For *M. bovis* (**pyruvate** is replaced by **glycerol**)

To Study the Characteristic Features of *Pseudomonas* spp.

Objective: Study colony characters of *Pseudomonas* species and preparation of smear and Gram staining, and study motility.

Colony Characteristics of Pseudomonas

Name of Media: Nutrient agar

1. Shape : Circular
2. Size : Large
3. Elevation : Flat
4. Surface : Smooth, glistening with a metallic sheen
5. Edge : Irregular
6. Consistency : Opaque
7. Emulsifiability : Easy
8. Pigment : Green colored diffusible pigment seen
9. Change in medium : Green colored due to diffusible pigment
10. Odor : Musty/earthy smell appreciated

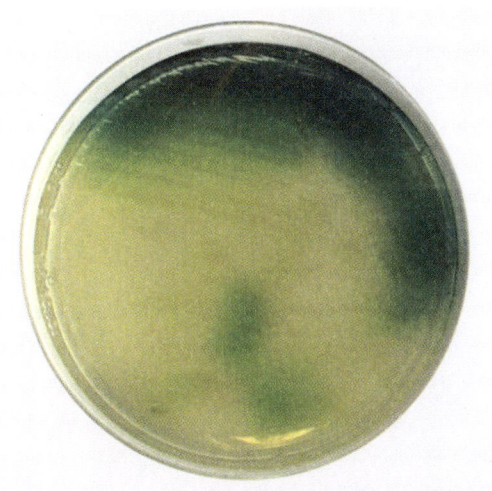

Green pigment producing colonies of Pseudomonas on nutrient agar

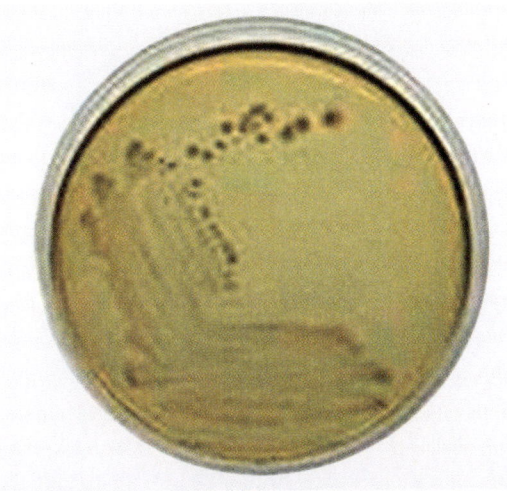

NLF colonies with characteristic musty/frooty odor are seen on MacConkey agar

Smear and Gram Staining

- Put a drop of normal saline in the middle of a clean grease-free glass slide.
- Make a smear of the colony provided, dry and heat fix the slide.
- Pour **crystal violet (primary stain)** on the smear and keep for 1 min.
- Decant the stain and pour **grams iodine (mordant)** on the smear.
- **Decolorize with acetone** for 2–3 seconds.
- Wash the slide and **counterstain with safranin** for 1 min.

Observation of Gram Stain of *Pseudomonas* spp.

Gram-negative bacilli are seen.

Observation of Motility of *Pseudomonas* spp. from the Broth Provided

Actively motile bacilli are seen.

Confirmatory Tests for *Pseudomonas* spp.

1. Catalase test—positive
2. Oxidase test—positive
3. Nitrate is reduced to nitrite
4. Oxidative utilization of sugars in OF media
5. Arginine dihydrolase test is positive.

Proteus spp.

Gram-negative bacilli are seen

Other Agents Causing Lower Respiratory Tract Infections, e.g. *Staphylococcus aureus, Pneumococcus, Aspergillus* spp. (Revision Practical)

Staphylococcus aureus

Gram-positive cocci are seen in clusters

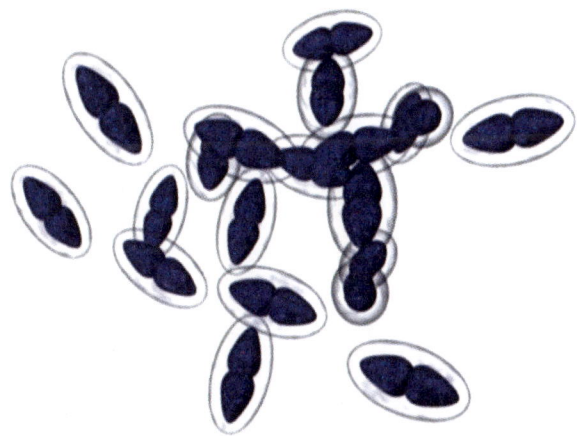

***Streptococcus pneumoniae* (pneumococci):** Gram-positive diplococci; Lanceolate/flame-shaped with wider ends adjacent.

207

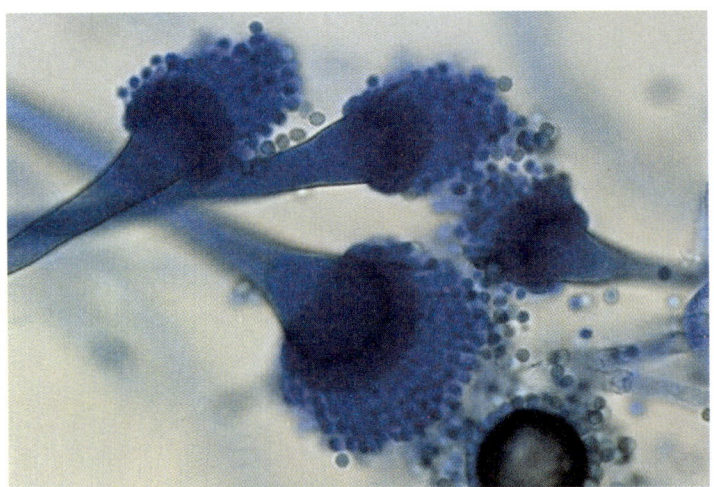

LPCB of *Aspergillus* spp.

Identify the Microbial Agents Causing Meningitis

Table of Agents Causing Meningitis

Agents Causing Meningitis

Type of agent	Name of agent	Age group	Method of detection	Detection feature
Bacteria	Eschrichia coli	Neonates and infants	Gram stain Culture	Gram-negative bacilli
	Haemophilus influenzae	Neonates and infants Young children	Gram stain Culture	Small gram-negative bacilli
	Neisseria meningitidis	Children adults	Gram stain Culture	Gram-negative diplococci
	Streptococcus pneumoniae	Neonates and infants Children, adults, elderly	Gram stain Culture	Gram-positive diplococci
	Streptococcus agalactiae	Neonates and infants	Gram stain Culture	Gram-negative cocci
	Staphylococcus aureus	Neonates and infants Elderly	Gram stain Culture	Gram-positive cocci in clusters
	Listeria monocytogenes	Older people, pregnant women, those with immune deficiency	Gram stain Culture	Gram-positive bacilli
	M. tuberculosis		ZN stain	AFB seen
	Klebsiella species	Neonates and infants	Gram stain Culture	Short thick gram-negative bacilli
Parasite	Acanthamoeba	Any age group	Wet mount Giemsa stain	Motile trophozoites Cysts
	Naegleria fowleri	Any age group	Wet mount Giemsa stain	Motile trophozoites Cysts
	Balamuthia mandrillaris	Any age group	Wet mount Giemsa stain	Motile trophozoites Cysts
	Toxoplasma gondii	Any age group	Serology	Antibody

Contd.

Contd.

Type of agent	Name of agent	Age group	Method of detection	Detection feature
Fungi	*Cryptococcus neoformans*	Immunodeficient HIV seropositives	India ink staining	Capsulated yeasts
	Candida albicans	Any age group	Wet mount Gram stain	Yeast cells Gram-positive budding yeast cells
	Histoplasma capsulatum	Any age group	Culture isolation Thermal dimorphism	LPCP stain after culture
	Coccidioides immitis	Any age group	Culture isolation Thermal dimorphism	LPCP stain after culture
Virus	*Coxsackie A and B*	Any age group	Serology PCR	Antibody Viral genome
	Echovirus	Any age group	Serology PCR	Antibody Viral genome
	Poliovirus	Any age group	Serology PCR	Antibody Viral genome
	West Nile virus	Any age group	Serology PCR	Antibody Viral genome
	Mumps	Any age group	Serology PCR	Antibody Viral genome
	Measles	Any age group	Serology PCR	Antibody Viral genome
	HIV	Any age group	Serology PCR	Antibody Viral genome
	Herpes simplex	Any age group	Serology PCR	Antibody Viral genome

Table to differentiate between bacterial/viral/fungal meningitis

	Normal	Bacterial	Viral	Fungal/TB
Pressure (cmH$_2$O)	5–20	>30	Normal of mildly increased	
Appearance	Normal	Turbid	Clear	Fibrin web
Protein (g/L)	0.18–0.45	>1	<1	0.1–0.5
Glucose (mmol/L)	2.5–3.5	<2.2	Normal	1.6–2.5
Gram stain	Normal	60–90% positive	Normal	
Glucose-CSF:Serum ratio	0.6	<0.4	>0.6	<0.4
WCC	<3	>500	<1000	100–500
Other		90% PMN	Monocytes 10% have >90% PMN 30% have >50% PMN	Monocytes

To Study the Characteristic Features of Gram-negative cocci *Neisseria meningitidis*

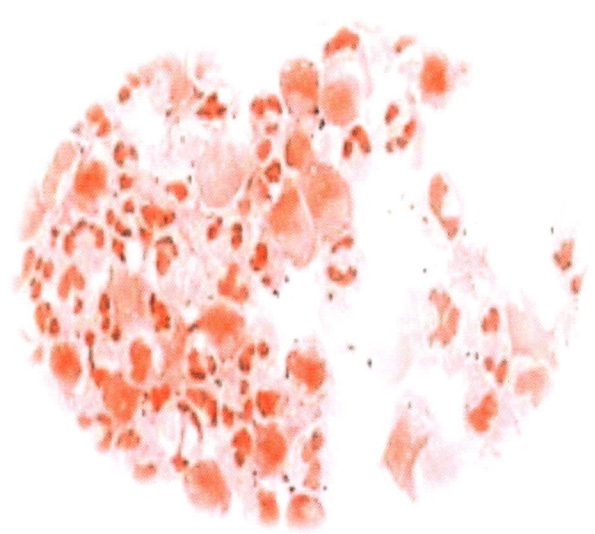

Capsulated gram-negative diplococci with adjacent sides flattened (*N. meningitidis*)

	N. gonorrhoea	*N. meningitidis*
Portal of entry	Genital tract	Respiratory tract
Polysaccharide capsule	Absent	Present
Beta-lactamase production	Some	None
Acid from maltose	Negative	Positive
Vaccine	Not available	Available

Other Agents Causing Meningitis, e.g. *Staphylococcus aureus*, *Streptococcus* spp., *E.coli*, *Klebsiella* spp., *M. tuberculosis* (Revision Practical)

Staphylococcus aureus: Gram-positive cocci are seen in clusters

Streptococcus pyogenes: Gram-positive cocci are seen in chains

Escherichia coli: Long thin gram-negative bacilli are seen

Klebsiella spp.: Short plump gram-negative bacilli are seen

Tubercular meningitis caused by the AFB *M. tuberculosis* on ZN staining of CSF

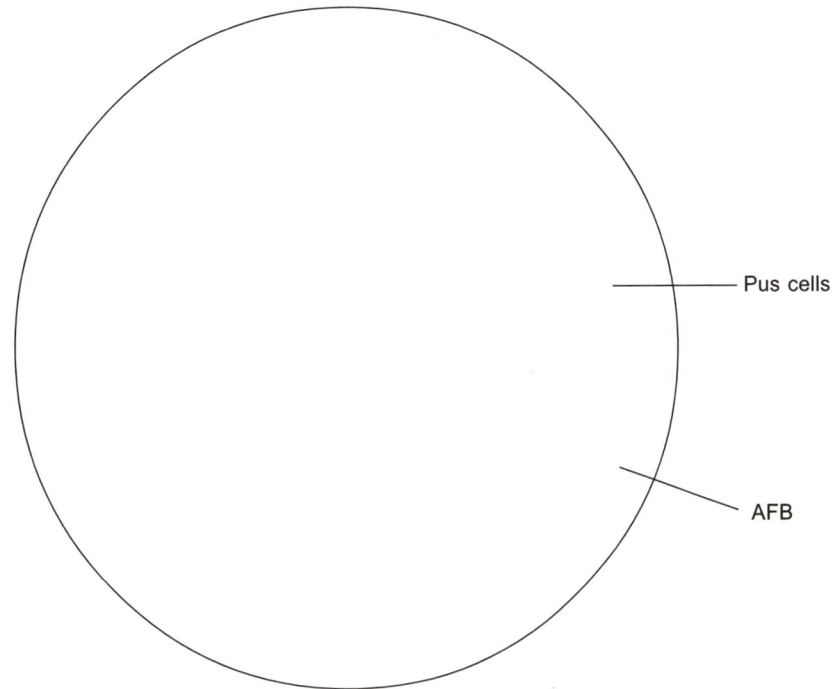

Pus cells

AFB

Cryptococcal meningitis—as seen in India Ink. preparation

Demonstrate Infection Control Practices and Use of Personal Protective Equipment (PPE)

Demonstration of Infection Control Practices

Objectives

- To elucidate the 5 moments of hand hygiene
- To demonstrate hand washing steps
- To show all PPE
- To demonstrate steps of donning and doffing of PPE.

The most important infection control practice is **hand hygiene.**

Why is hand hygiene so important?

The most common way germs (bacteria, viruses, parasites, fungi) are spread by hands. Germs cannot only cause illnesses such as colds, flu, typhoid, diarrheal diseases, hepatitis A/E, but accusation of multi-drug resistant bacteria MRSA or ESBL producing GNBs, etc. can lead to health care associated infections. Simply touching a patient or his surrounding objects can transfer these organisms to the hands of health care workers (HCWs) and then gets transferred to another patient leading to cross-contamination and spread of health care associated infections. Hand hygiene is the most effective and also the cheapest way to prevent such infections and is the main infection control practice. Use soap and water preferably or using hand rub containing at least 70% ethyl alcohol.

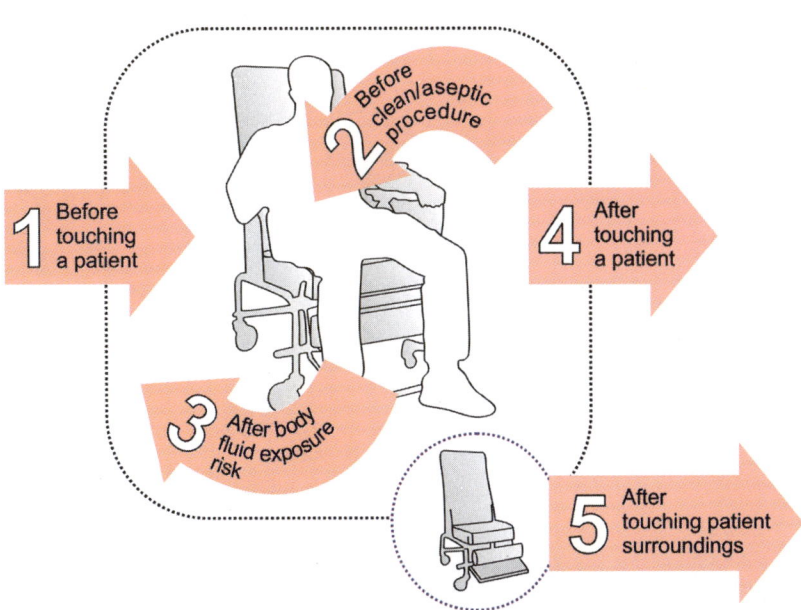

Your 5 moments for hand hygiene
Source: https://openwho.org/courses/IPC-HH-en

229

Mnemonic for Hand Washing/Hygiene Steps (SUMAN-K)

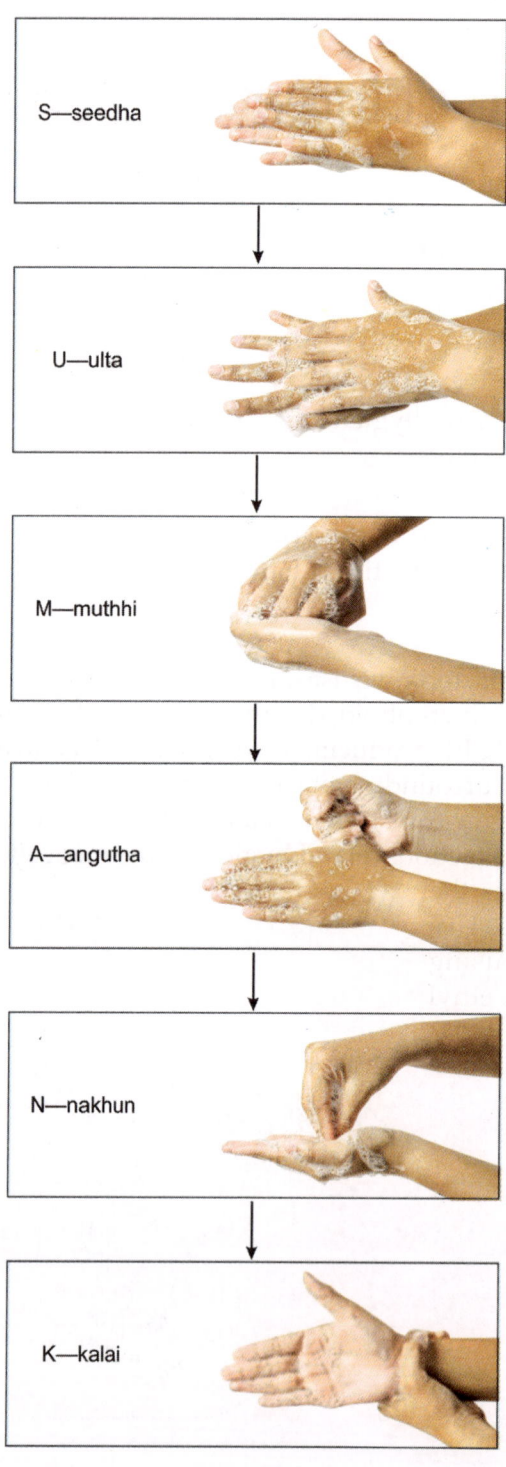

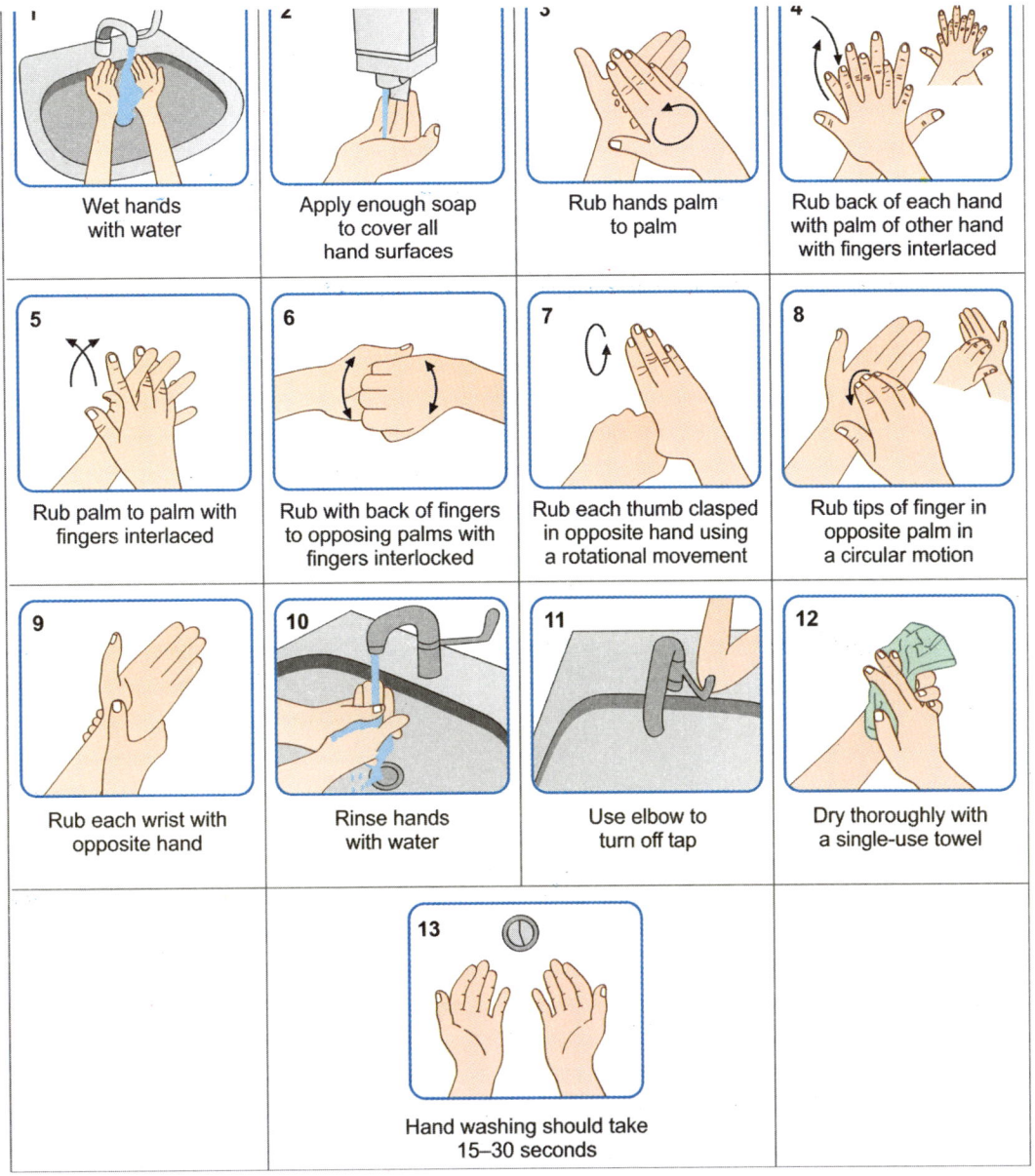

Hand washing technique with soap and water

Source: https://www.pinterest.com/pin/400257485634424486/

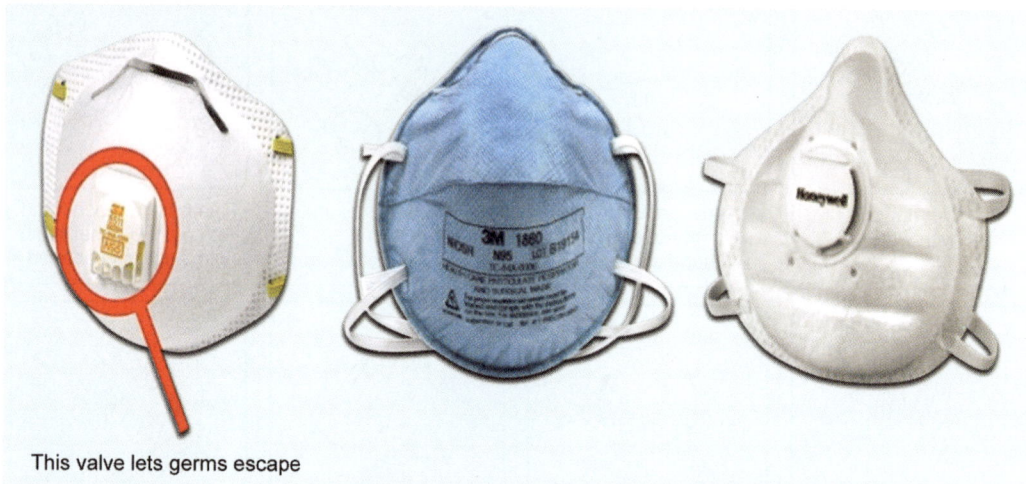

This valve lets germs escape

N-95 masks with valves NOT to be used

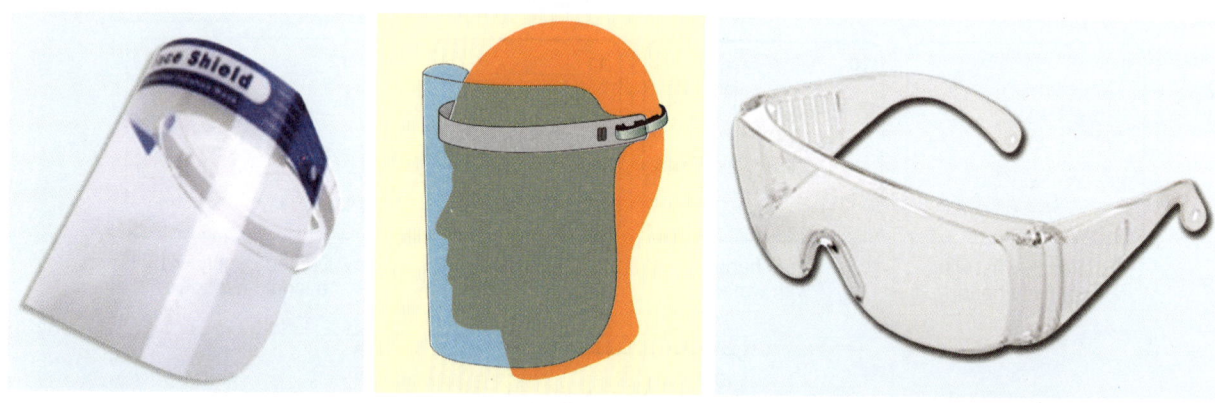

Face-shield   PPE goggles

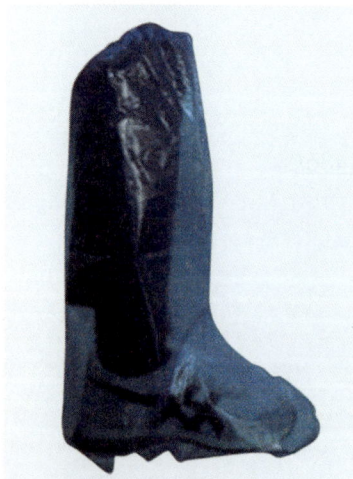

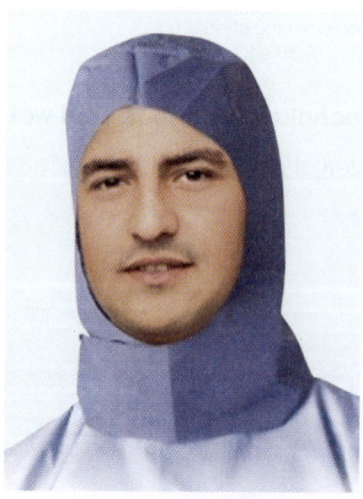

PPE shoe cover   PPE head cover

Personal Protective Equipment (PPE)

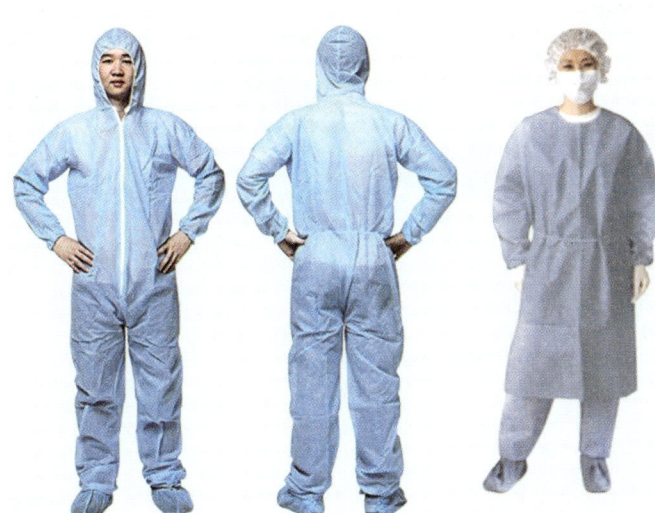

- Coverall/gown—**fiber or plastic**
- Three-ply surgical **mask** or N-95 masks without valve
- Goggles and face-shields
- Gloves/face-shield
- **Shoe covers**
- **Head covers**

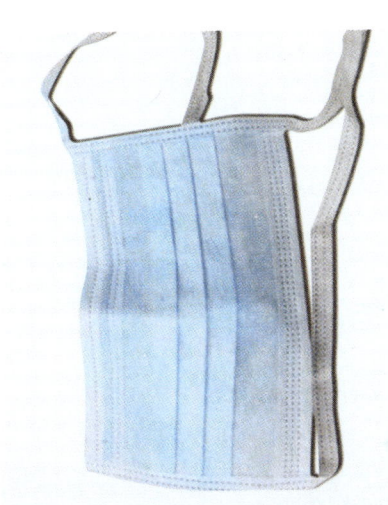

3-ply surgical mask

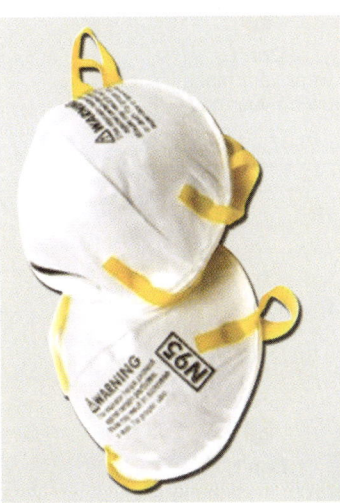
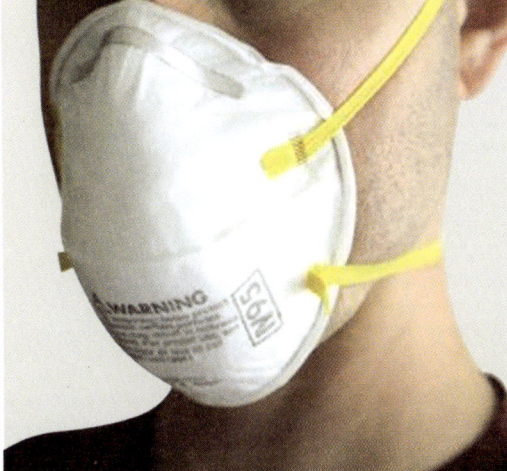

N-95 mask

233

The mask conundrum

The centre has written to all states and Union Territories warning against the use of N-95 masks with valve respirators, saying these do not prevent the virus from spreading

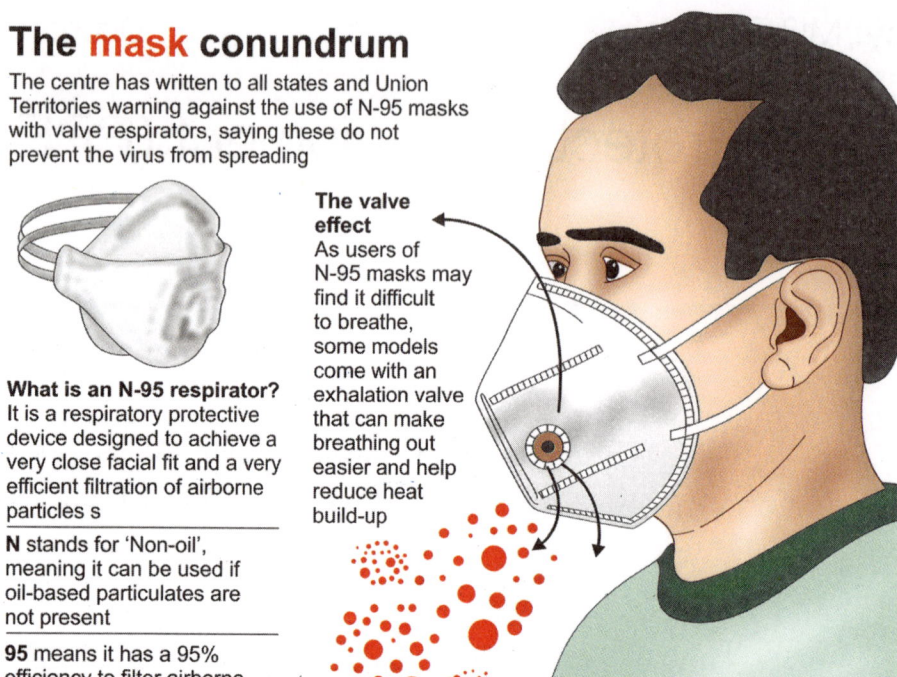

What is an N-95 respirator?
It is a respiratory protective device designed to achieve a very close facial fit and a very efficient filtration of airborne particles s

N stands for 'Non-oil', meaning it can be used if oil-based particulates are not present

95 means it has a 95% efficiency to filter airborne particles

The valve effect
As users of N-95 masks may find it difficult to breathe, some models come with an exhalation valve that can make breathing out easier and help reduce heat build-up

Always wash hands before and after wearing your mask and clean resuable masks after use. Avoid touching the mask at all times and only use the bands or ties to put on and remove.

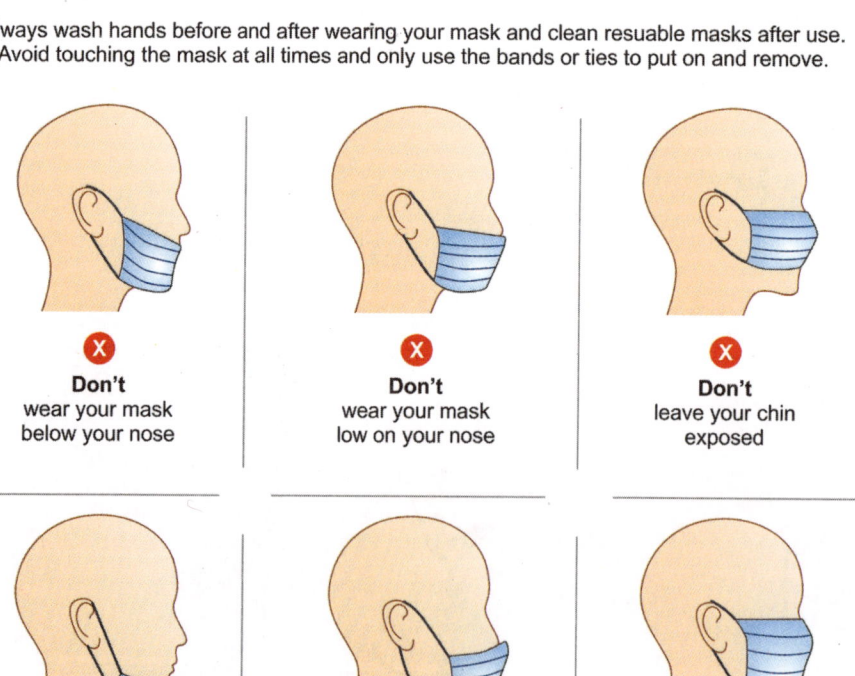

❌ **Don't**
wear your mask below your nose

❌ **Don't**
wear your mask low on your nose

❌ **Don't**
leave your chin exposed

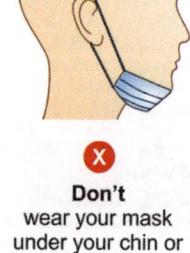

❌ **Don't**
wear your mask under your chin or temporarily remove it in public

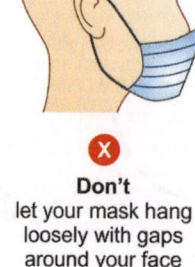

❌ **Don't**
let your mask hang loosely with gaps around your face

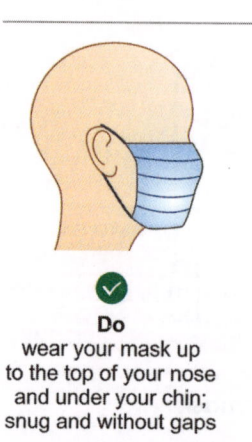

✅ **Do**
wear your mask up to the top of your nose and under your chin; snug and without gaps

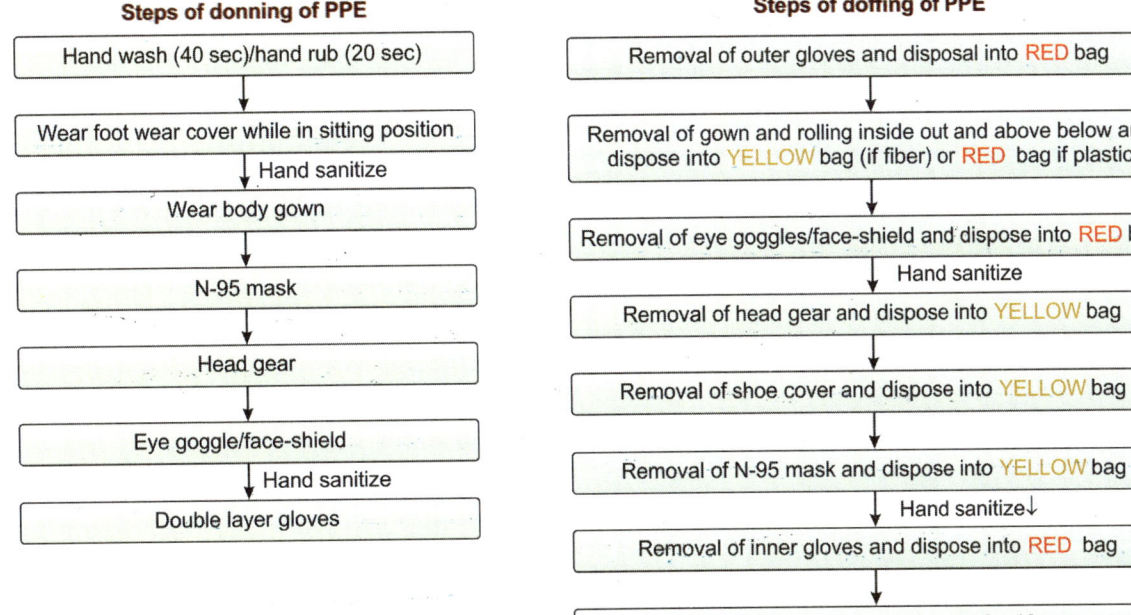

Steps of donning of PPE

Hand wash (40 sec)/hand rub (20 sec)

Wear foot wear cover while in sitting position

Hand sanitize

Wear body gown

N-95 mask

Head gear

Eye goggle/face-shield

Hand sanitize

Double layer gloves

Steps of doffing of PPE

Removal of outer gloves and disposal into RED bag

Removal of gown and rolling inside out and above below and dispose into YELLOW bag (if fiber) or RED bag if plastic

Removal of eye goggles/face-shield and dispose into RED bag

Hand sanitize

Removal of head gear and dispose into YELLOW bag

Removal of shoe cover and dispose into YELLOW bag

Removal of N-95 mask and dispose into YELLOW bag

Hand sanitize↓

Removal of inner gloves and dispose into RED bag

Hand wash with soap and water for 40 sec

Removing gown

- Unfasten ties
- Peel gown away form neck and shoulder
- Turn contaminated outside toward the inside
- Fold or roll into a bundle and discard

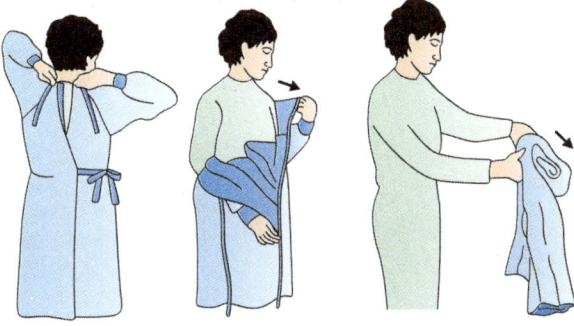

Demonstrate the Appropriate Method of Collection of Samples in the Performance of Laboratory Tests in the Detection of Microbial Agents Causing Infectious Diseases

52. Specimens and Collection
- Demonstrate Method of Collection of Blood Samples from Children and Adults
- Demonstrate Method of Inoculation of Blood for Blood Culture in the Detection of Microbial Agents Causing Septicemia
- Amount, Number and Type of Blood Cultures
- Transport and Incubation of Blood Culture Bottles
- How to Minimize Contamination in Blood Culture
- Other Types of Microbiological Specimens Used for Detection of Microorganisms Causing Infectious Diseases
- Criteria for Rejection of a Microbiological Sample
- Transport and Storage of Microbiological Samples when Delay in Transport and Testing
- Various Microbiology Specimens with Respect to Type of Infection

Specimens and Collection

Demonstrate the appropriate method of collection of samples in the performance of laboratory tests in the detection of microbial agents causing infectious diseases.

Learning Objectives

- Method of collection of blood samples from children and adults.
- How to inoculate blood for blood culture?
- Amount, number and type of blood cultures.
- Transport and incubation of blood culture bottles.
- How to minimize contamination?
- Other types of microbiological specimens used for detection of microorganisms.
- Criteria for rejection of a sample.
- Transport and storage of samples when delay in transport and testing.

Principles of Specimen Management

It is important to know relevant requirements for specific specimens and diagnostic protocols for infectious disease diagnosis.

1. The laboratory must follow a standard operating procedure (SOP).
2. A specimen should be collected prior to administration of antibiotics. Once antibiotics have been started, the microflora changes, leading to potentially misleading culture results.
3. Specimens must be labeled accurately and completely so that interpretation of results will be reliable. Labels such as "eye" and "wound" are not helpful to the interpretation of results without more specific site and clinical information (e.g. dog bite wound right forefinger).
4. Microbiology specimens should be delivered to the testing laboratory without delay, and follow specific instructions for specimen transport and stability.
5. Many body sites have normal flora that can easily contaminate the specimen. Therefore, specimens from sites such as lower respiratory tract (sputum), nasal sinuses, superficial wounds, fistulae, and others require care in collection.
6. The laboratory requires a specimen, not a swab for collection of a specimen. Tissue, aspirates, and fluids are always specimens of choice, especially from surgery. A swab is not the specimen of choice for many specimens because swabs pick up extraneous microbes, hold extremely small volumes of the specimen (0.05 ml), make it difficult to get bacteria or fungi away from the swab fibers and onto media, and the inoculum from the swab is often not uniform across several different agar plates. However, nasopharyngeal and oropharyngeal swabs are processed for viral respiratory infections.

7. Specimens of poor quality must be rejected.

8. Physicians should not demand that the laboratory report "everything that grows," thus providing irrelevant information that could result in inaccurate diagnosis and inappropriate therapy.

9. Susceptibility testing should be performed on clinically significant isolates, not on all microorganisms recovered in culture.

General principles for all specimen collection

1. Standard precautions should be followed for handling and collection all types of specimens.

2. All specimens should be collected in sterile leak proof containers.

3. All specimens for microbiological culture should preferably be collected before the start of antimicrobials.

4. Actual tissue, aspirates, and body fluids are always specimens of choice compared to swabs.

5. All specimens should be appropriately labelled after collection before it reaches the lab.

Various Microbiology Specimens with Respect to Type of Infection

Type of infection	Specimen to be collected
Sepsis /BSI/endocarditis	Blood culture
URTI	Throat swab (nasopharyngeal/oropharyngeal)
LRTI	Sputum (gastric aspirate in children), ETA, BAL, PSB, pleural fluid, lung biopsy
UTI	Voided midstream urine, catheter sample, suprapubic aspirate
Diarrheal disease	Stool, rectal swab
Skin and soft tissue infections	Pus/exudates, wound swab, tissue biopsy, aspirates
CNS infections	CSF
Eye infections	Aqueous/vitreous tap, corneal scrapings, conjunctival swab
Ear infections	Pus/discharge swabs
Reproductive/genital tract infections	Uretheral/high vaginal swab, cervical cytobrush, exudates from genital ulcers, Tzank smear, endometrial curettage
Serology	Whole blood
Malaria	Peripheral blood smear, anticoagulated blood for Ag
Filariasis	Peripheral blood smear after DEC provocation test
Kala-azar	Bone marrow smear
Bone and joint infections	Pus/discharge, sequestrum, synovial fluid
Superficial fungal infections	Skin scraping, nail clippings, scalp scraping, proximal one cm hair with hair root
Rabies	Biopsy from nape of neck, corneal impression smear, postmortem brain impression smear

1. **Specimens and collection for bloodstream infection (BSI)**
2. **Procedure for collection of blood sample by venipuncture**

- Identify the patient and note patient's details on the vial before collection.

- Patient to be seated on a chair. Wear sterile gloves.

- Keep needle and syringe ready, air should be expelled from syringe completely.

- Tie a tourniquet 2–3 inches distal to the venipuncture site.

- Ask patient to make a fist so that veins become prominent.

- Palpate the antecubital fossa (preferred site for venipuncture) for prominent vein.

- Disinfect the venipuncture site (center to periphery in a circular manner) first with 70% isopropyl alcohol → air dry → then applying 2% chlorhexidine. Disinfection with tincture of iodine (or 10% povidone iodine; chlorhexidine not recommended for children <2 months old) requires 1 minute of air dry time once disinfection is completed. *Vein should not be palpated after disinfection unless a gloved finger is also disinfected.*

- Hold the patient's arm and place the left thumb below the venipuncture site.

- Enter the needle into the vein swiftly at 30° angle and withdraw 5–10 ml blood depending on the number of tests to be done.

- Once sufficient blood has collected, release the tourniquet before withdrawing the needle.

- Give the patient a clean gauze pad to keep the punctured area covered with gentle pressure.

- Transfer the blood immediately into desired vial (in case of EDTA vial invert the sample in the vial 2–3 times to mix properly with the additive.

- Destroy the needle in the needle cutter and dispose hub with syringe in red bin.

- Once no more blood comes out from venipuncture site the gauze can be disposed and a band-aid applied.

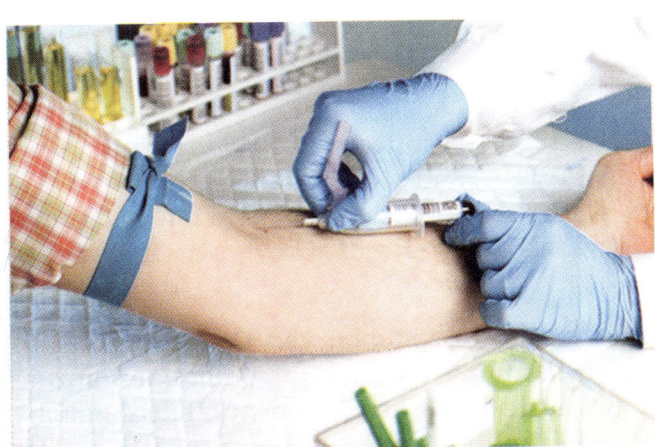

5 ml syringe with needle

16–18 gauze needle in adults

22 gauze needle in children

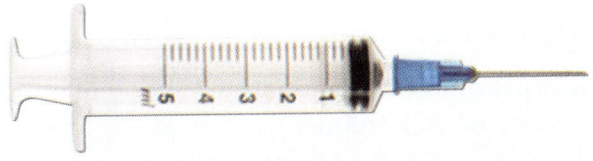

Amount of blood: At least 1–3 ml whole blood collected aseptically by venipuncture, preferably before the initiation of antimicrobial therapy and inoculated directly into pediatric blood culture bottle containing 20–25 ml broth for blood culture. For adults 5–10 ml blood in 45–50 ml broth is recommended. The ratio is approximately 1 part blood in 9 parts broth (1:9). In case of patients on antimicrobial therapy *plus* aerobic (BACTEC) automated blood culture bottles can be used. Once blood is transferred to culture bottles, invert the bottles gently to prevent clotting.

Types of blood culture: If both **aerobic and anaerobic blood cultures** are required specific bottles for this purpose will have to be inoculated separately. To decide which bottle is to be inoculated first, if using a winged blood collection set then the aerobic bottle should be filled first to prevent transfer of air in the device into the anaerobic bottle. If using syringe needle inoculate the anaerobic bottle first to avoid entry of air. If the amount of blood drawn is less than the recommended volume, then aerobic bottle should be inoculated first with the required volume of blood, since most of the bacteremia are caused by the aerobic facultative bacteria. In addition, pathogenic yeasts and strict aerobes (e.g. *Pseudomonas*) are recovered almost exclusively from aerobic bottles. Any remaining blood should then be inoculated into the anaerobic bottle.

   Mycobacterial culture acid-fast bacilli (AFB) specific BC bottles are to be used.

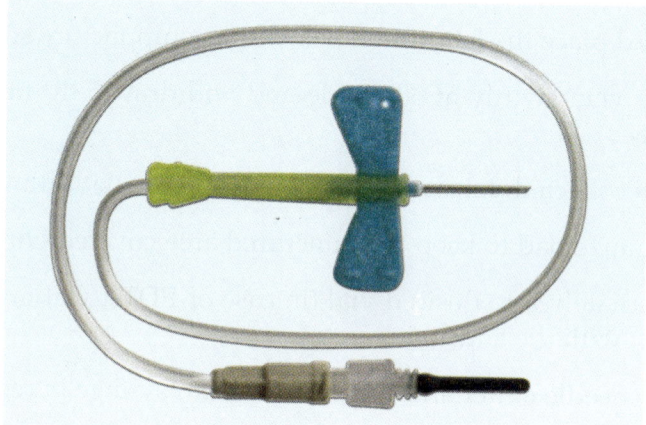

Winged blood collection set

Number of blood cultures: In case of acute bacterial endocarditis, at least three sets of blood cultures (BCs), separated from one another by at least 1 hour, should be obtained from separate venipuncture sites before initiation of antibiotic therapy. In cases of suspected subacute bacterial endocarditis, obtain 3 BCs on the first day, spacing the venipuncture at least 30 minutes apart. If these are negative, obtain 2 more sets on subsequent days.

   In case of **pyrexia of unknown origin** (PUO) and suspected **fungal septicemia**, blood to be inoculated in a biphasic BC bottle containing brain heart infusion agar (BHIA) and broth (BHIB). If PUO, two BCs can initially be drawn with an interval of 45–60 minutes. The reason for the time interval is to determine if a continuous or intermittent bacteremia exists. Two more sets of BCs can then be drawn 24–48 hours later if necessary.

How to minimize contamination? Skin contaminants in BC bottles are common, very costly to the health care system, and frequently confusing to clinicians. To minimize the risk of contamination, the venipuncture site and rubber septum of BC bottles require disinfection. The venipuncture site should be

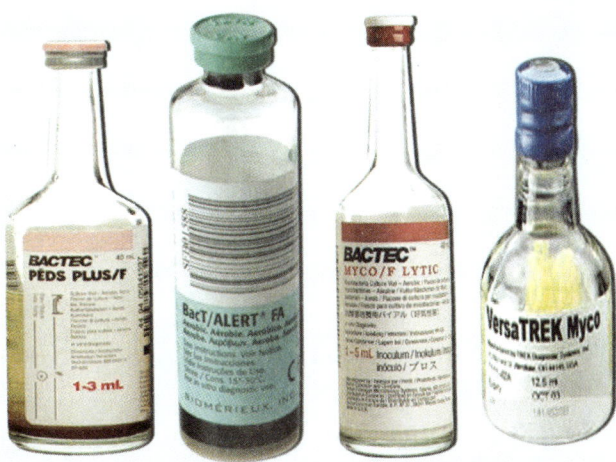

Different automated blood culture bottles

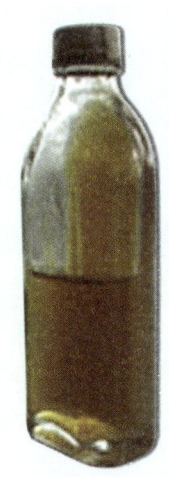

Biphasic blood culture bottle

cleansed (center to periphery in a circular manner) first with 70% isopropyl alcohol, air dried, and then the main disinfectant applied. Disinfection with tincture of iodine (or 10% povidone iodine; chlorhexidine not recommended for children <2 months old) requires 1 minute of air dry time once disinfection is completed. *Vein should NOT be palpated after disinfection unless the gloved finger is also disinfected.* The rubber septum on the BC bottle(s) should be decontaminated with 70% isopropyl alcohol, which can be allowed to air dry while venipuncture is performed.

Clot cultures are more productive in yielding better results in isolation as it overcomes the lower sensitivity of BCs attributed to the low concentration of bacteria circulating in blood (<15 organisms/ml and the bactericidal action of serum is also obviated. Blood after clotting has to be lysed either mechanically with sterile glass beads or with streptokinase which may be expensive in developing countries.

Transport and incubation of blood culture bottles: Bottles should be transported immediately to the laboratory. In case of delay bottle(s) to be kept at 37°C in incubator in case of manual BCs/kept at RT (22–25°C) in case of automated BCs (BACTEC) for a maximum of 24 hours.

Whole blood/serum may also be sent for serological tests like C-reactive protein, rheumatoid factor, VDRL/RPR, Widal test, various bacterial/parasitic/viral antibody (Ab), antigen (Ag) detection by rapid point of care (POC) tests/ELISA.

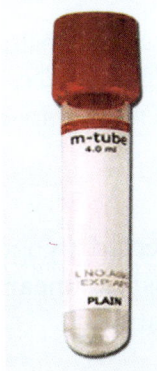

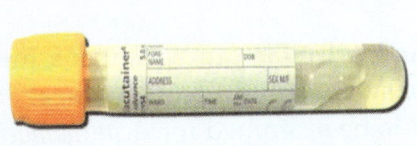

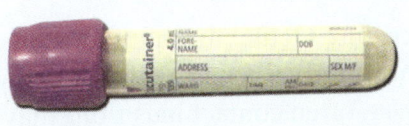

Plain vial (red cap) and with gel (yellow cap) for whole blood to obtain serum.
EDTA vial (purple cap) for anticoagulated blood

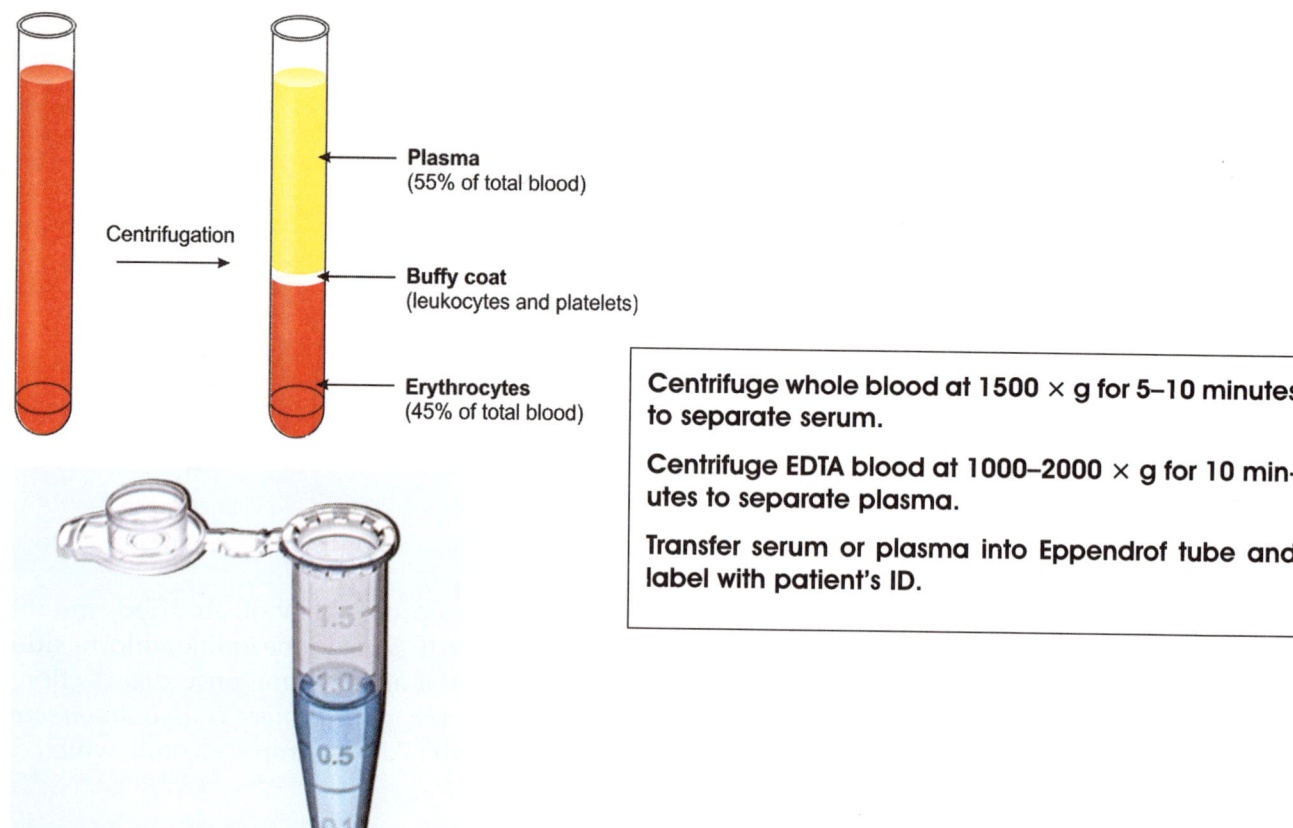

Centrifuge whole blood at 1500 × g for 5–10 minutes to separate serum.

Centrifuge EDTA blood at 1000–2000 × g for 10 minutes to separate plasma.

Transfer serum or plasma into Eppendrof tube and label with patient's ID.

A **bone marrow aspirate** should be sent immediately preferably after informing the laboratory or smears can be made on glass slides.

Central nervous system infections—CSF sample to be obtained by lumbar puncture and sent to microbiology, biochemistry and cytology laboratory. A minimum of 0.5–1 ml of CSF should be sent immediately after collection to the microbiology laboratory in a sterile container for bacterial/parasitic/viral testing. Sample for microbiology laboratory to be stored at room temperature and not in refrigerator in case of delay in transport as suspected *Haemophilus influenzae* is very sensitive to low temperatures.

A wet mount prepared for probable fungus, motile trophozoites or cysts of parasites like free living amoeba (*Acanthamoeba, Naegleria, Balamuthia*). India Ink. preparation for *Cryptococcus*.

Gram stain is done (by heaped up method if CSF is not visibly turbid) for presence of gram-positive/gram-negative bacteria (e.g. *Escherichia coli, Haemophilus influenzae, Neisseria meningitidis, Streptococcus pneumoniae, Staphylococcus aureus, Listeria monocytogenes*) pus cells or yeast cells (e.g. *Candida* species, *Cryptococcus neoformans*).

Giemsa stain for parasites.

Ocular infections: Ocular fluids like **aqueous and vitreous tap** specimens for suspected pyogenic infections, **conjunctival swab, corneal scrapings, swabs from ulcers, corneal impression smear** for suspected *rabies*, often contact lens fluid may need to be examined for *Acanthamoeba* keratitis.

Eye samples are almost always collected by ophthalmologists. The volume of specimens is always limited. This specimen limitation makes it necessary for the laboratory to prioritize procedures depending on what organisms are sought; this should always be done after discussion with the ophthalmologists. Specimens should be labeled with the specific anatomic source, i.e. conjunctiva or cornea, but not just "eye."

Upper and lower respiratory infections (URTI/LRTI): A **throat swab** (moistened with sterile normal saline) swabbing both side the fauces, pillars and lastly the posterior pharyngeal wall should be taken from the oropharynx in case of URTI. Deep coughed out **sputum** and not saliva collected in a sterile wide mouth container, **bronchoalveolar lavage** (BAL) and **tracheal aspirate** are the specimens for LRTI. A **plural fluid** aspirate can also be used for laboratory analysis. In case the child is not able to cough out, cough may be induced by nebulized hypertonic saline. In case of very small child **gastric aspirate** may suffice as the child normally swallows the sputum.

In case of suspected respiratory viral infections including COVID-19 infection, a **nasopharyngeal and oropharyngeal swab** (NPS and OPS) sample is taken and immediately immersed in viral transport medium (VTM), swirled in the VTM and the extra part of the swab projecting out of the VTM container is broken off, lid of VTM closed and transported on ice as soon as possible to the microbiology laboratory. A flocked/dacron/rayon swab is preferable than cotton swabs for viral infections. Flocked swabs are more effective than even dacron, or rayon swabs as it allows for more efficient release of contents for evaluation.

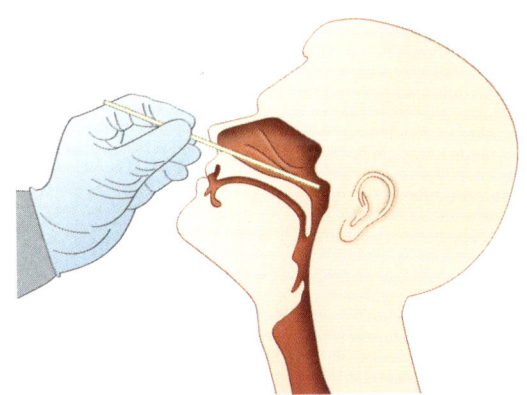

NPS collection

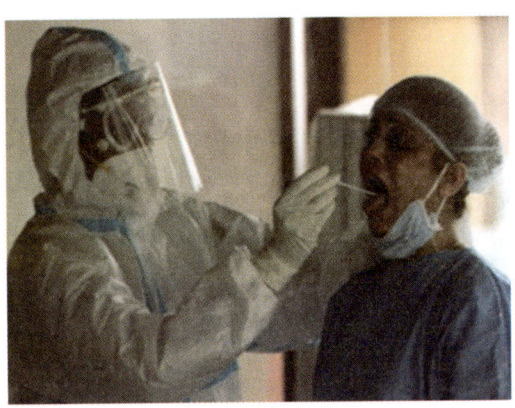

OPS collection

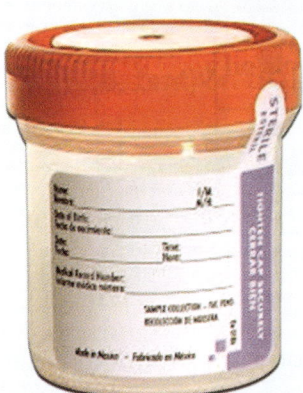

Sterilized wide mouth universal container

Sputum collection: Early morning sputum sample to be collected in wide mouth sterile container. BACTEC NAP vials are recommended for mycobacterial cultures

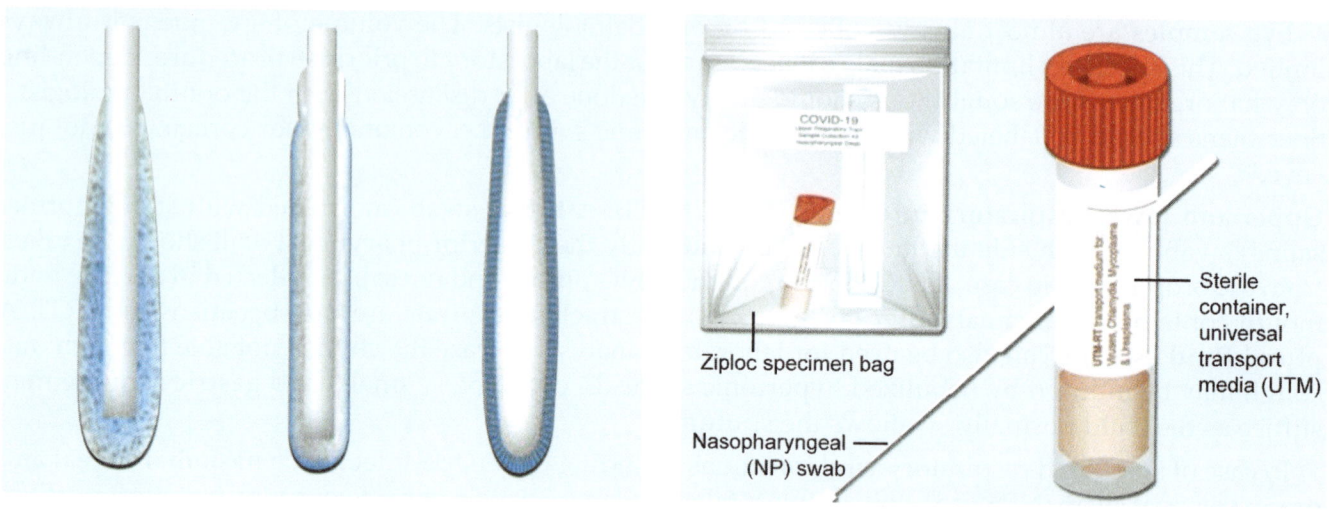

Flocked swabs

Swab with VTM

Skin and soft tissue infections—tissue biopsy to be sent in normal saline; **purulent exudates** or **discharge** from wound, surgical sites, lesions can either be sent in moist swab or needle aspirated and sent in sterile vial depending upon the quantity; **aspirate** of any skin lesion like blister fluid can be sent in VTM and transported on ice for suspected viral etiology or in sterile vial for bacterial etiology.

For suspected anaerobic infections, the wound should be cleaned first to remove the superficial contaminating aerobes and then samples of discharge or needle aspirate should be taken from the depth of the wound and immediately transferred in anaerobic medium like thioglycollate medium/Robertson's cooked meat broth (RCM) and then transported to the laboratory. Swabs are unsatisfactory. Avoid contact with oxygen, avoid refrigeration and preferably to be processed soon after collection.

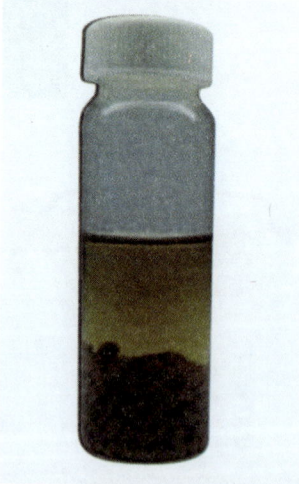

Robertson's cooked meat broth (RCM)

Skin scraping, nail clippings, proximal 1–2 cm of **hair** including hair root (after shampooing) for superficial fungal infections should be collected on kraft paper using a sterile scalpel after patient has been instructed to withhold application of any skin/head ointment for 24 hours and the area has been washed with soap and water and dried. For mycetoma, the lesion should be covered by a sterile moist gauge and left overnight and the gauge should be sampled the following day to track the discharging grains.

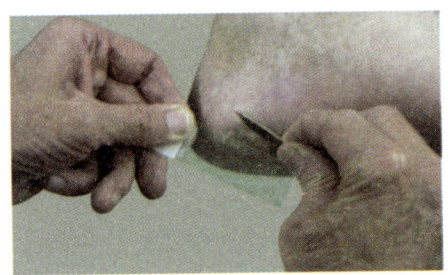
Skin scraping

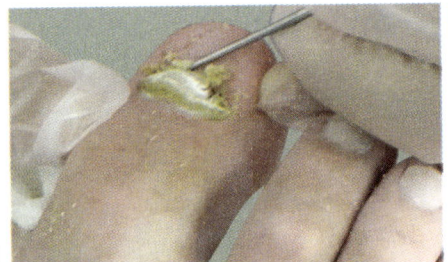
Nail scraping/clipping

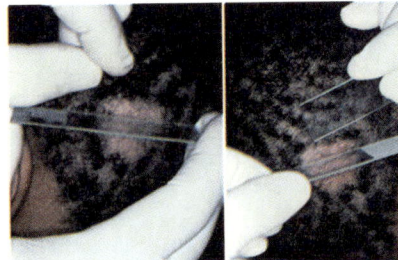
Sampling of hair/scalp

Gastrointestinal (GI) and intra-abdominal infection—stool sample (preferable) or **rectal swab** in case of gastroenteritis to be collected in a clean wide mouth universal container, **string test sample** for Giardiasis, **biopsy** material from duodenum, jejunum, colon are to be sent in sterile vial in normal saline. **Vomitus or leftover food** may be sent in case of food poisoning. **Ascitic/peritoneal fluid, pus from liver abscess** are other important samples. Stool samples should be transported as early as possible after collection to retain motility of trophozoites.

For rectal swab, insert swab at least 2.5 cm beyond the anal sphincter so that it enters the rectum and rotate it once before withdrawing. Transport in Cary and Blair semisolid transport medium.

Bone and joint infections: Sequestrum, bone chip, immersed in normal saline/in TGB (for anaerobic culture), **pus** from osteomyelitis, **synovial fluid,** to be sent to laboratory for processing (thioglycollate broth).

Urinary tract infections: After a holding period of 4 hours, voided clean catch midstream urine sample (10 ml approximately) is to be collected in a wide mouth sterile leak proof universal container after proper genital toileting with nonmedicated soap and clean water and then dried with a towel. If patient is catheterized then sample should be taken from catheter tube after clamping below the collection port so that urine can collect in the catheter tubing in 15–20 minutes. Then after disinfecting the catheter above the collection port, 5–10 ml of urine sample is aseptically collected with needle and syringe. Urine is never collected and not from urobag. Sample is to be labelled as catheterized sample.

In suprapubic needle aspiration urine is collected directly from bladder and is preferred in infants, and in patients whom anaerobic bacteria resuspected as cause of UTI.

Genital infections: High vaginal swab or **endocervical swab** collected by gynecologists and sent in sterile test tube to the lab. Exceptionally in case of ulcerative lesions a **Tzank smear, pus** from genital chancre/**urethral discharge. Biopsy** in case of genital warts may be sent.

After introduction of warm moist vaginal speculum, and wiping away excess mucus, the swab or cervical brush is inserted deep into the vagina and rotated there before withdrawing it.

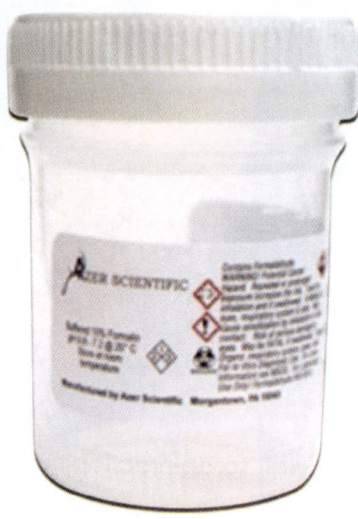

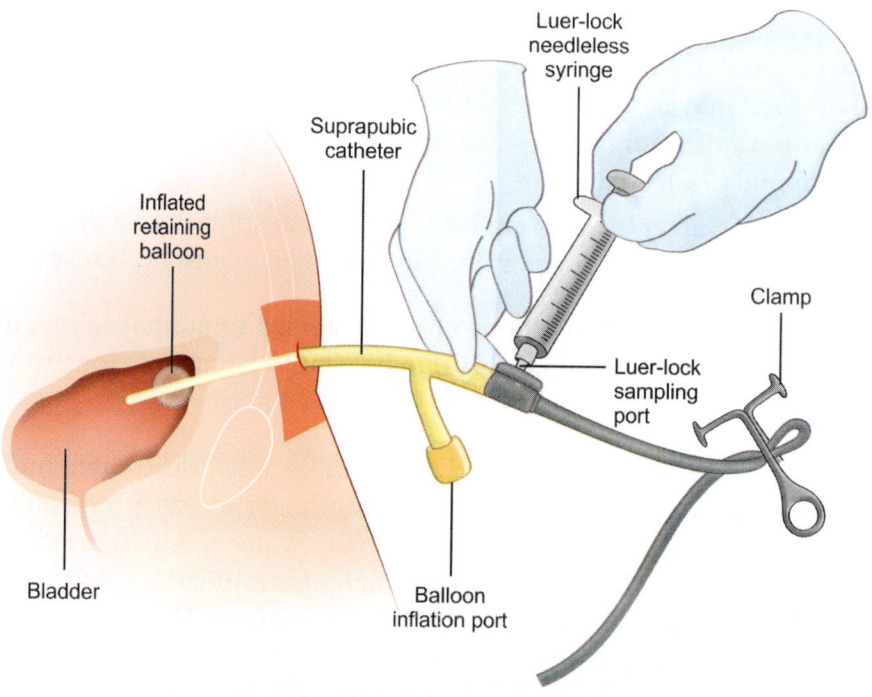

Sterile universal container

Quality of Specimen

Specimens of poor quality would have to be rejected to avoid inaccurate diagnosis and inappropriate therapy. Specimens from sites such as lower respiratory tract (sputum), nasal sinuses, superficial wounds, fistulae, etc. require care in collection as their indigenous flora can easily contaminate the inappropriately collected specimen and complicate interpretation.

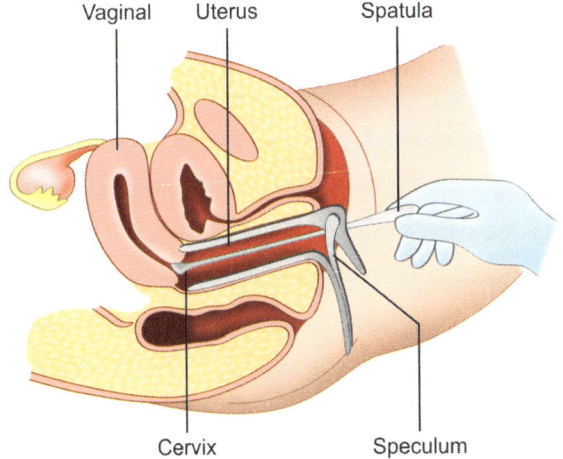

Vaginal   Uterus   Spatula

Cervix   Speculum

After introduction of warm moist vaginal speculum, and wiping away excess mucus, the swab or cervical brush is inserted deep into the vagina and rotated there before withdrawing it.

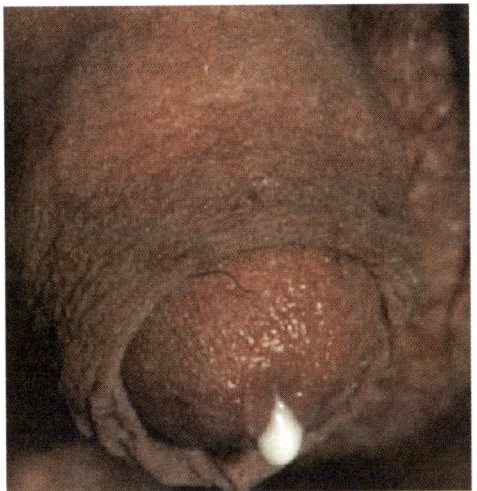
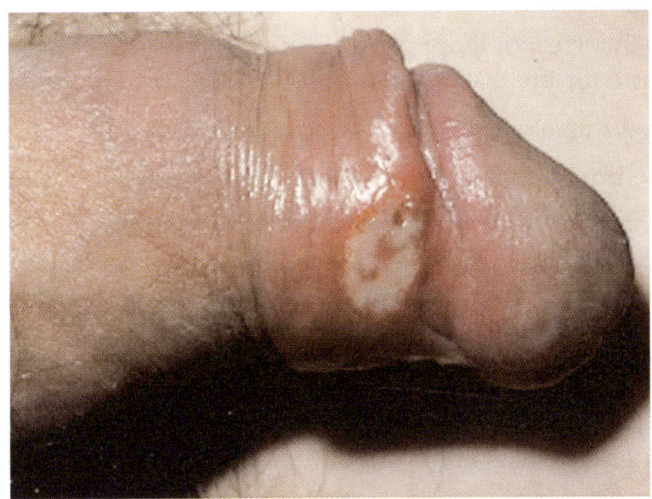

Pus from urethral discharge/genital chancre

Actual tissue, aspirates, and fluids are always specimens of choice compared to swabs because swabs pick up extraneous microbes, hold extremely small volumes of the specimen (0.05 ml), and make it difficult to get bacteria or fungi away from the swab fibers and onto media, and the inoculums from the swab is often not uniform across several different agar plates. Swabs are expected from the nasopharynx and to diagnose most viral respiratory infections.

- A specimen should be collected prior to administration of antibiotics.
- Once antibiotics have been started, the microbiota changes and etiologic agents are impacted, leading to potentially misleading culture results.
- Susceptibility testing should be done only on clinically significant isolates.
- Accurate and complete labeling of specimens allows reliable interpretation of results.
- Close communication between the clinician and the microbiologist is essential to ensure that appropriate specimens are selected and collected and that they are appropriately examined.

Criteria for sample rejection

1. Unlabelled or improperly labelled samples

2. Samples in leaky containers are unacceptable when the outside of the container is grossly contaminated with the sample. In this case, request a new sample.

3. Contaminated samples are unacceptable. In the case of a contaminated sample, request a new sample.

4. Inappropriate sample sources

   Samples that do not conform to the type of sample needed for the requested test(s) are unacceptable.

   - For example:
     - Do not process saliva in place of sputum.
     - 24-hour urine samples are unacceptable for routine bacterial cultures.
     - The type of anticoagulant for a blood sample (or the absence of an anticoagulant) must be appropriate for the type of blood test.

   - If an incorrect or inappropriate sample type is received, request a new sample and specify the proper sample for the test requested.

5. Delayed transport time and sample processing

   - If the time between sample collection and receipt is too long for a valid test to be performed, with respect to sample requirements for the requested test(s), request a new sample.

   - If a sample was received after prolonged delay but is not rejected by the laboratory, document it and indicate the length of time after collection that the sample was received.

Actions for when samples are rejected

- If the unacceptable sample can be replaced, notify the requesting health care provider.

- Document the reason for the sample unacceptability and request another sample.

- Do not discard the sample until the patient's health care provider has confirmed that another can be collected.

   If a repeat sample is not available, document the problem and proceed with the test if possible.

Storage of samples in case of delay in transport to lab

Sample	Storage temperature
• Serum	4–8°C refrigerator
• Blood culture bottle (manual)	37°C incubator
• BACTEC blood culture bottle	Room temperature (22–25°C)
• CSF	Room temperature (22–25°C)
• Urine, stool, body fluids	4–8°C refrigerator
• Samples for fungus	4–8°C refrigerator

Storage of serum samples before testing. For <7 days at 4–8°C; For >7 days at –20°C/–80°C

Packaging of samples for transport

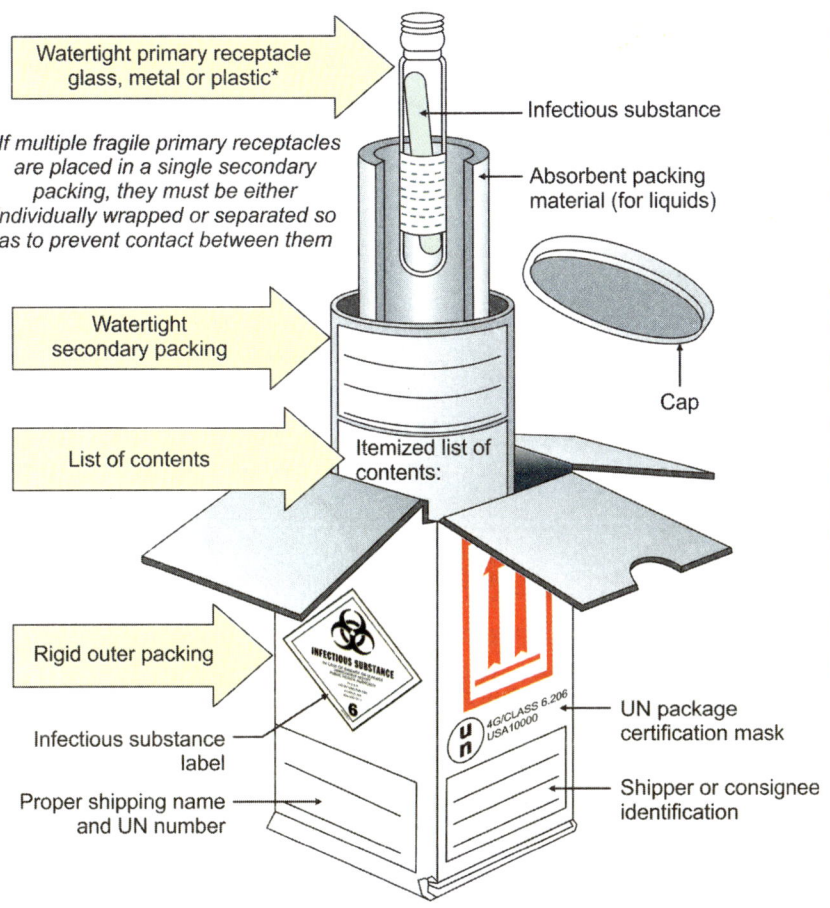

Watertight primary receptacle glass, metal or plastic*

If multiple fragile primary receptacles are placed in a single secondary packing, they must be either individually wrapped or separated so as to prevent contact between them

Watertight secondary packing

List of contents

Rigid outer packing

Infectious substance
Infectious substance label

Proper shipping name and UN number

Absorbent packing material (for liquids)

Cap

Itemized list of contents:

UN package certification mask

Shipper or consignee identification

- **Primary container:** Sample in leak proof container. Tightly capped surrounded by absorbent material.

- **Secondary container:** The primary container is put into a water tight leak-proof secondary container. Several primary containers can be put in one secondary container. Each should be labelled. Additional absorbent material should be put to cushion the primary containers.

- **Outer container:** Secondary container is put in the rigid outer box. Ice packs if required can be put here. Outer box should contain complete address and a biohazard label.

Section
12

Demonstrate Respect for Patient Samples Sent to the Laboratory for Performance of Laboratory Tests in the Detection of Microbial Agents Causing Infectious Diseases

53. To be able to Demonstrate Need for Confidentiality Pertaining to Patient Identity with Regards to Laboratory Results

Demonstrate Confidentiality Pertaining to Patient Identity in Laboratory Results

Demonstrate respect for patient samples sent to the laboratory for performance of laboratory tests in the detection of microbial agents causing infectious diseases.

Confidentiality is the right of an individual to have personal, identifiable medical information kept private. Such information should be available only to the physician of record and other health care and insurance personnel as necessary. Because the disclosure of personal information could cause professional or personal problems, patients rely on physicians to keep their medical information private.

Doctors have an ethical and legal duty to respect patient confidentiality. This means that personal and medical information given to a health care provider will not be disclosed to others unless the individual has given specific permission for such release which requires doctors to seek consent "where practicable", and to inform patients about the use of their data keeping their identity anonymous. Creating thorough policies and confidentiality agreements, providing regular training and making sure all information is stored on secure systems are some of the other ways to maintain patient confidentiality.

It is rare for medical records to remain completely sealed, however. The most benign breach of confidentiality takes place when clinicians share medical information as case studies. When this data is published in professional journals the identity of the patient is never divulged, and all identifying data is either eliminated or changed. If this confidentiality is breached in any way, patients may have the right to sue.